DORLAND'S GASTROENTEROLOGY SPELLER

Consultant

SIDNEY COHEN, MD
Richard Laylord Evans Professor of Medicine
Chairman, Department of Medicine
Temple University School of Medicine
Philadelphia, Pennsylvania

Consultant for Syllabication

CAROL A. HART, PhD
Narberth, Pennsylvania

DORLAND'S GASTROENTEROLOGY SPELLER

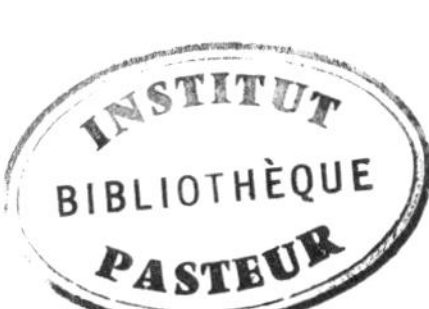

W.B. SAUNDERS COMPANY
A Division of Harcourt Brace & Company
Philadelphia London Toronto Montreal Sydney Tokyo

W. B. SAUNDERS COMPANY
A Division of
Harcourt Brace & Company

The Curtis Center
Independence Square West
Philadelphia, Pennsylvania 19106

Library of Congress Cataloging-in-Publication Data

Dorland's gastroenterology speller.

p. cm.

ISBN 0–7216–4568–2

1. Gastroenterology—Terminology. I. W. B. Saunders Company. II. Title: Gastroenterology speller. [DNLM: 1. Gastroenterology—nomenclature. 2. Gastrointestinal Diseases—nomenclature. WI 15 D711]

RC802.D67 1993 616.3′3′0014—dc20

DNLM/DLC 92–13353

Dorland's Gastroenterology Speller ISBN 0–7216–4568–2

Printed in the United States of America

Last digit is the print number: 9 8 7 6 5 4 3 2 1

Preface

Dorland's Gastroenterology Speller continues the task set by previous Dorland's spellers, that is, to provide a comprehensive list of terms within a health care specialty, since, as has been noted in the previous spellers, the entire body of medical vocabulary is much too large to include in a single volume. As always, acceptable end-of-line breaks have been given, and multiple listings for hard-to-find terms, such as proper names and trademarks, have been given.

The word list has been compiled from a number of sources, including the *Dorland's Illustrated Medical Dictionary* database and a variety of texts, monographs, and journals in gastroenterology. Also included are terms from the official Latin nomenclature. Special attention has been given to difficult terms, such as eponyms and trademarks.

Thanks are owed to Sidney Cohen, MD, who reviewed the word list, and to Carol A. Hart, PhD, who provided the hyphenation. Their efforts have been extremely helpful in making this a comprehensive and authoritative reference.

DOUGLAS M. ANDERSON
Chief Lexicographer

How This Book Is Arranged

Order of Entries

Dorland's Gastroenterology Speller follows the same scheme of arrangement as *Dorland's Illustrated Medical Dictionary*. Main entries follow one another in letter-by-letter alphabetical order regardless of spaces or hyphens that occur within them (see below for special rules for chemical names); compound entries consisting of one or more adjectives and a noun will be found as subentries under the noun. In some cases where there might be a question about where to look to find an entry, entries have been given in more than one place, even under an adjective.

Eponymic terms. Terms containing a proper name are given multiple listings, once under the thing named and once under each eponym. Thus *Richner-Hanhart syndrome* is listed as:

syndrome
  Richner-Hanhart s.
Hanhart
  Richner-H. syndrome
Richner
  R.-Hanhart syndrome

Umlauts are ignored for alphabetization, and proper names beginning *Mc* or *Mac* are alphabetized as though spelled *Mac*.

Chemical prefixes. Italicized chemical prefixes such as the letters *p*- and *o*- and *cis*- and *trans*-, together with numbers, Greek letters, and the small capitals L- and D-, do not count for alphabetization. When prefixes are written out in full, however, as *para*- instead of *p*-, they are counted for alphabetical order.

Subentries

Each subentry appears on a new line following the main entry and is indented. The main entry word in a subentry is represented only by the initial letter (as *duodenal p.* under *papilla*), with three exceptions. For regular English plurals, the abbreviation is the initial letter followed by *'s* (as *t's* for *tests*). For irregular or Greek or Latin plurals, the entire plural form is written out (as *venae* under *vena*). For possessive forms, the initial letter is followed by *'s* (as *G's diverticulum* for *Ganser's diverticulum*. In subentries the main entry word is ignored for alphabetization, as are prepositions, conjunctions, and articles.

Possessive Forms

The use of the possessive in eponyms is controversial. This book follows the example of *Dorland's Illustrated Medical Dictionary,* that is, the *'s* is favored where the sources for a term justify its appearance. Whether or not to use the possessive form is a matter left to the individual; owing to the present lack of consistency and consensus, no prescription can be given.

Abbreviations and Acronyms

A number of abbreviations and acronyms are given, together with the words or phrases that they stand for. The selection is of course only a small fraction of the abbreviations and acronyms in actual use. If more than one word or phrase is listed with an abbreviation, the terms are given in alphabetical order and each additional term is placed on a new line and indented.

Word Divisions

Acceptable word divisions are given for main entries; syllabication is based on pronunciation. Not all syllable breaks are shown; for example, because single letters at the beginnings and ends of words may not be separated from the rest of the word, such divisions are not given. Likewise, single letters should not be separated from the word elements they belong to in compound words. Breaks that could confuse the reader as to the meaning of a word are to be avoided. In many cases, words may be broken at other places than the ones that appear in this book (for example, different pronunciations imply different word breaks); it is impossible to show every break that could occur for every word. What appears here is one possible system.

Alternative Spellings

A number of words have alternative spellings, ranging from the difference of a single letter to the use of variant forms of Greek and Latin stems. Although every effort has been made to ensure that the spellings included in this book are valid, no indications of preference are given.

Brackets and Parentheses

Some entries require a bit of explanation; these explanations are enclosed in parentheses. Brackets are sometimes used as a part of Latin anatomical nomenclature to enclose an eponym in the genitive case; in this book such eponyms generally appear all lower case (as in *Dorland's Illustrated Medical Dictionary)* but an initial capital for the name is acceptable.

Plurals

Plurals for foreign words, all of them Greek and Latin, are given with the appropriate entries. In addition, they are given again as separate entries if they do not occur within a few lines of the singular form.

Contents

A

A
albumin
antrectomy

AAC
antibiotic-associated pseudomembranous colitis

Aagen•aes
A. syndrome

AAOC
antacid of choice

AAPC
antibiotic-associated pseudomembranous colitis

AAPMC
antibiotic-associated pseudomembranous colitis

AB
abdominal

Ab•bott
A. esophagogastrostomy
A.-Miller tube
A.-Rawson tube
Miller-A. tube

ABCRS
American Board of Colon and Rectal Surgery

ABD
abdomen
abdominal

Abd
abdomen
abdominal

abd
abdomen
abdominal

abdo
abdomen
abdominal

ABDOM
abdomen
abdominal

Abdom
abdomen
abdominal

abdom
abdomen
abdominal

ab•do•men
acute a.
pendulous a.
surgical a.

ab•dom•i•no•per•i•ne•al

abeta•lipo•pro•tein•emia

A bile

Abi•plat•in

ABM
adjusted body mass

Abrams
Gilman-A. gastric tube

ab•scess
amebic a.
appendiceal a.
appendicular a.
bile duct a.
biliary a.
cholangitic a.
diverticular a.
epiploic a.
fecal a.
helminthic a.
hepatic a.
interloop a.
intersphincteric a.
intramesenteric a.

ab•scess *(continued)*
intraperitoneal a.
ischiorectal a.
pancreatic a.
pararectal a.
pelvic a.
pelvirectal a.
perianal a.
pericolic a.
peritoneal a.
pyogenic a.
stercoraceous a.
stercoral a.
subphrenic a.

Ab•sid•ia
A. capillata

absorp
absorption

ab•sorp•ti•om•e•try
dual photon a.

ab•sorp•tion
enteral a.
intestinal a.

AbSR
abdominal skin reflexes

abuse
laxative a.

ABV
doxorubicin, bleomycin sulfate, and vinblastine

ABVD
doxorubicin, bleomycin sulfate, vinblastine, and dacarbazine

ABW
actual body weight

AC
abdominal circumference
abdominal compression
activated charcoal
acute cholecystitis
alcoholic cirrhosis

a.c.
L. ante cibum (before meals)

Acan•tho•ceph•a•la

acan•tho•cy•to•sis

ac•an•tho•sis
glycogenic a.

ACBE
air-contrast barium enema

ACD
adult celiac disease

ac•et•al•de•hyde

acet•a•min•o•phen
a., sodium bicarbonate, and citric acid

ac•et•a•zol•a•mide

ac•e•tor•phine

acet•y•la•tion

ac•e•tyl•cho•line

ac•e•tyl•cho•lin•es•ter•ase

ac•e•tyl co•en•zyme A

ac•e•tyl•cys•te•ine

5-ac•e•tyl•sal•i•cyl•ic ac•id

ac•e•tyl•trans•fer•ase

ACG
American College of Gastroenterology

ach•a•la•sia
pelvirectal a.

achlor•hy•dria

achlor•hy•dric

acho•lan•gic

acho•lia

acho•lic

achol•uria

achol•uric

Achro•my•cin V

achy•lia

ac•id
- 5-acetylsalicylic a.
- amino a.
- aminolevulinic a.
- 4-aminosalicylic a.
- arachidonic a.
- ascorbic a.
- chenodeoxycholic a.
- cholic a.
- citric a.
- dehydrocholic a.
- fatty a.
- hyaluronic a.
- α-keto a.
- linoleic a.
- oleic a.
- retinoic a.
- secondary bile a.
- short chain fatty a.
- sialic a.
- uric a.
- ursodeoxycholic a.
- valproic a.

ac•id hy•dro•lase

ac•i•do•sis
- lactic a.

aci•nus *pl.* aci•ni
- hepatic a.
- liver a.
- pancreatic acini

ac•i•vi•cin

ACL
- anal canal length

ac•la•cin•o•my•cin A

Ac•me One Time en•ter•al feed•ing bag

ACMI en•do•scope

ACMI fi•ber•op•tic proc•to•sig•moido•scope

ACMI gas•tro•scope

ACMI T-915 fi•ber•op•tic sig•moido•scope

ACMI TX-915 fi•ber•op•tic sig•moido•scope

acop•ro•sis

acop•rous

Ac•ta-Char

Ac•ti•dose

Ac•ti•gall

ac•tiv•i•ty
- specific a.

acy•clo•vir

Ad
- adipocyte

Adair
- A. tissue holding forceps
- Allis-A. tissue forceps

Ad•ams
- Mayo-A. self-retaining appendectomy retractor

Ad•ap•in

ad•ap•ta•tion
- intestinal a.

ADC
- antral diverticulum of the colon

ADE
- apparent digestive energy

ad•e•ni•tis
- mesenteric a.
- phlegmonous a.

ad•e•no•car•ci•no•ma
- esophageal a.

ad•e•no•ma
- Brunner's gland a.
- colorectal a.
- hepatic a.
- hepatocellular a.
- liver cell a.

ad•e•no•ma *(continued)*
multiple a's
serrated a.
tubular a.
tubulovillous a.
villous a.

ad•e•no•myo•epi•the•li•o•ma
a. of stomach

ad•e•no•my•o•ma

ad•e•no•my•o•ma•to•sis

aden•o•sine

ad•e•no•vi•rus

ad•he•sion
bacterial a.
cell a.

ad•he•sive
tissue a.

ad•i•po•cele

ad•i•po•he•pat•ic

ad•i•po•sis
a. hepatica

ADP
advanced pancreatitis

ad•re•ner•gic

adre•no•cor•ti•coid
glucocorticoid a's

Adri•a•my•cin

Adri•a•my•cin PFS

Adri•a•my•cin RDF

Adru•cil

Ad•son
A. dissecting hook
A. forceps
A. needle holder
A. suction tube
A.-Brown forceps

AEP
acute edematous pancreatitis

Aero•mo•nas
A. hydrophila

Aero•plast

aer•o•sol
hydrocortisone acetate rectal a.

AES
anterior esophageal sensor

AF
ascitic fluid

Af•ko-Lube

AFLP
acute fatty liver of pregnancy

AGA
American Gastroenterological Association

agas•tria

agas•tric

AGE
acute gastroenteritis

agent
alkylating a.
contrast a.
iodinated contrast a.
oral contrast a.
water-soluble contrast a.

ag•gre•ga•tion
bile salt a.

Ag•or•al

AGS (gastric cancer) cell

AH
acute hepatitis
alcoholic hepatitis

AHR-9294 (H^+ pump inhibitor)

A-hydro•Cort

AIDS
 acquired immunodeficiency syndrome

AJCC/UICC stag•ing (for colorectal carcinoma)

Aj•ma•lin
 A. liver disease

Ala•gille
 A's syndrome

Al•a•mag

al•a•nine

al•a•nine ami•no•trans•fer•ase

Alax•in

al•ben•da•zole

Al•bert
 A's suture
 A.-Lembert suture

al•bu•min

al•de•hyde de•hy•dro•gen•ase (NAD^+)

al•do•ster•one

ALF
 acute liver failure

al•fax•a•lone

al•fen•ta•nil

Al•fer•on N

Al•gen•ic Al•ka

Al•gi•con

al•ka•line phos•pha•tase

al•ka•li•ther•a•py

al•ka•lo•sis

Al•ka-Mints

Al•ka-Selt•zer

Al•ker•an

Al•len
 A. cecostomy trocar
 A. intestinal clamp
 A.-Kocher clamp

al•ler•gy
 food a.

Al•lis
 A. clamp
 A. forceps
 A. tissue forceps
 A.-Adair tissue forceps
 Duval-A. tissue forceps
 Judd-A. intestinal forceps
 Thoms-A. tissue forceps

Al•li•son
 A. repair

al•lo•pur•i•nol

All-Sil•i•cone Side-Eye EFT feed•ing tube

Al•ma•cone

Al•ma•cone II

Al•ma-Mag Im•proved

Al•ma-Mag #4 Im•proved

al•oe
 cascara sagrada and a.

Al•o•phen

al•pha$_1$-an•ti•tryp•sin

Al•pha•mul

al•pha 2,6-si•al•yl•trans•fer•ase

AL•ter•na•GEL

Al•tra•cin

Alu-Cap

Alu•drox

alu•mi•na
a. and magnesia
a. and magnesium carbonate
a. and magnesium trisilicate
a., magnesia, and calcium carbonate
a., magnesia, and simethicone
magnesium trisilicate, a., and magnesia
a., magnesium trisilicate, and sodium bicarbonate
simethicone, a., calcium carbonate, and magnesia

alu•mi•num
basic a. carbonate
a. hydroxide

Alu-Tab

amas•ti•gote

am•a•tox•in

ame•ba *pl.* ame•bae, ame•bas

ame•bi•a•sis
hepatic a.
intestinal a.

ame•bic

ame•bi•ci•dal

ame•bi•cide

Amer•i•can di•la•tor

Amer•i•can En•dos•co•py litho•trip•tor

Amer•i•can Gas•tro•en•ter•o•log•i•cal As•so•ci•a•tion

Amer•i•can So•ci•ety for Gas•tro•in•tes•ti•nal En•dos•co•py

A-metha•Pred

am•i•ka•cin

Am•i•kin

amil•o•ride

Amin-Aid re•nal for•mu•la

ami•no acid
branched-chain a.a.
nonessential a.a's

ami•no•lev•u•lin•ic acid

ami•no•pep•ti•dase

4-ami•no•sal•i•cyl•ic ac•id

ami•no•thi•a•da•zole

ami•no•trans•fer•ase

ami•o•da•rone

Am•i•tone

am•i•trip•ty•line

am•mo•nia

am•mo•ni•um
tetramethyl a.

Am•o•gel PG

amox•i•cil•lin
a. and clavulanate

Amox•il

AMP
adenosine monophosphate

3′5′-AMP
cyclic adenosine monophosphate

Am•pho•jel

amp•i•cil•lin
a. and sulbactam

Am•pi•cin

am•pul•la *pl.* am•pul•lae
duodenal a.
a. duodeni
hepatopancreatic a.
a. hepatopancreatica
Lieberkühn's a.
phrenic a.
rectal a.

am•pul•la *(continued)*
a. recti
a. of Vater

AMSA
amsacrine

Amsa
amsacrine

am•sa•crine

Am•ster•dam
A. stent

Amus•sat
A's operation

am•y•lase
serum a.

am•y•lin

am•y•loi•do•sis
hepatic a.

AN
anorexia nervosa

an•acid•i•ty
gastric a.

ANAD
anorexia nervosa and associated disorders

anal

anal•y•sis *pl.* anal•y•ses
image a.
near-infrared reflectance a.
3-day stool a.

ana•phy•lax•is
intestinal a.

an•a•scit•ic

Ana•spaz

an•a•stal•sis

an•as•to•mo•sis *pl.* an•as•to•mo•ses
antecolic a.
antiperistaltic a.

an•as•to•mo•sis *(continued)*
biliary-enteric a.
Braun's a.
chole-enteric a.
coloanal a.
end-to-end a.
end-to-side a.
Gambee a.
gastrointestinal a.
Halsted a.
Hofmeister a.
ileal pouch–anal a.
ileocolic a.
ileorectal a.
ileosigmoid a.
intestinal a.
isoperistaltic a.
Navy single-layer everting a.
portacaval a.
primary a.
retrocolic a.
Polya a.
Roux-en-Y a.
Schoemaker a.
side-to-side a.
stapled a.
stapled end-to-end ileoanal a.
transanal a.

An•ca•lix•ir

an•chor
Cope viscerotomy a.

An•cy•los•to•ma
A. americanum
A. duodenale

an•cy•lo•sto•mat•ic

an•cylo•stome

an•cy•los•to•mi•a•sis

An•drews
A. suction tip

an•ep•i•plo•ic

An•er•gan

an•eu•rysm
cirsoid a.
extravisceral a.
gastric a.
intramural a.

an•gi•na
abdominal a.
a. abdominalis
a. abdominis
a. dyspeptica
intestinal a.

an•gio•dys•pla•sia
colonic a.
submucosal endothelial a.
submucosal fibromuscular a.

an•gio•gram

an•gi•og•ra•phy

an•gi•o•ma
gastric a.

an•gi•o•ma•to•sis
hepatic a.

an•gio•ten•sin
a. II

An•gio•vist

an•gle
anorectal a.
inferior a. of duodenum
superior a. of duodenum

an•gu•lus *pl.* an•gu•li
a. of stomach

an•hy•drase
carbonic a.

an•hy•dro•chlo•ric

an•ic•ter•ic

an•ion
organic a.

an•i•sa•ki•a•sis

An•i•sa•kis
A. marina

an•is•mus

an•iso•tro•pine

an•nu•lus *pl.* an•nu•li
a. femoralis
a. haemorrhoidalis
a. lymphaticus cardiae

Ano•col

ano•derm

anom•a•ly
Dieulafoy a.
a. of Zahn

ano•plas•ty
V-Y a.

ano•rec•tal

ano•rec•ti•tis

ano•rec•to•co•lon•ic

ano•rec•tum

an•orex•ia
a. nervosa

ano•scope
Bacon a.
Bodenheimer a.
Boehm a.
Brinkerhoff a.
Buie-Hirschman a.
Fansler a.
Ferguson a.
Goldbacher a.
Hirschman a.
Ives a.
Muer a.
Otis a.
Pratt a.
Pruitt a.
Sims' a.

An•son
A.-McVay femoral herniorrhaphy

AN-Sul•fur Col•loid

ant•ac•id

An•ta-Gel

An•ta•Gel-II

an•tag•o•nist
- CCK a.
- cholecystokinin a.
- interleukin-1 receptor a.
- KSG-504 CCK a.
- L-364,718 CCK a.
- L-365,260 CCK a.

an•throne
- rhein a.

an•ti•bi•ot•ic

an•ti•body
- antiendothelial cell a.
- indium In 111 murine anti-CEA monoclonal a. ZCE 025
- monoclonal a's

an•ti•en•do•the•li•al

an•ti•fi•lar•i•al

An•ti•flux

an•ti•gen
- adenoma-associated a.
- anti-40KDa colonic a.
- carcinoembryonic a. (CEA)
- hepatitis a.
- 40KDa colonic a.
- liver membrane a.
- liver-specific a.
- proliferating cell nuclear a. (PCNA)
- sialosyn-Tn a.
- squamous cell carcinoma a.

anti-HAA
- antibody to hepatitis-associated antigen

anti-HAV
- antibody to hepatitis A virus

anti-HB_SAg
- antibody to hepatitis B surface antigen

an•ti-HBc
- antibody to hepatitis B core antigen

anti-HBe
- antibody to hepatitis B e antigen

an•ti-HBs
- antibody to hepatitis B surface antigen

anti-HCV
- antibody to hepatitis C virus

anti-HDV
- antibody to hepatitis D virus

anti-40KDa

an•ti•mes•en•ter•ic

an•ti•neo•plas•tic

an•ti•ox•i•dant
- dietary a.

an•ti•per•i•stal•sis

an•ti•per•i•stal•tic

an•ti•plas•min
- α_2-a.

an•ti•pro•to•zo•al

an•ti•py•rine

an•ti•schis•to•so•mal

An•ti•spas

α_1-an•ti•tryp•sin

An•tre•nyl

An•tro•col

an•tro•du•o•de•nec•to•my

an•tro•py•lo•ric

an•trum *pl.* an•tra
cardiac a.
a. cardiacum
gastric a.
a. pylori
pyloric a.
a. pyloricum
a. of Willis

anus
artificial a.
ectopic a.
imperforate a.
preternatural a.
a. vesicalis
a. vestibularis
vulvovaginal a.

anus•i•tis

An•u•sol

An•xan•il

aor•ta *pl.* aor•tae, aor•tas
abdominal a.
a. abdominalis

aor•to•du•o•de•nal

aor•to•en•ter•ic

aor•to•esoph•a•ge•al

aor•to•gas•tric

AP
abdominoperineal
adenomatous polyp
appendectomy
appendix

a&p
abdominal and perineal

apan•crea

apan•cre•at•ic

APC
adenomatous polyposis coli

aper•i•stal•sis

apha•gia

aph•e•re•sis
T cell a.

aph•thous

Apo-Ami•trip•ty•line

Apo-Amoxi

Apo-Am•pi

Apo-Chlor•ax

Apo-Chlor•di•az•e•pox•ide

Apo-Ci•met•i•dine

Apo-Eryth•ro

Apo-Eryth•ro-ES

Apo-Eryth•ro-S

Apo-Hy•droxy•zine

apo•lipo•pro•tein

Apo-Me•tro•ni•da•zole

apo•neu•ro•sis *pl.* apo•neu•ro•ses
ischiorectal a.

apo•pro•tein

ap•op•to•sis

Apo-Ra•ni•ti•dine

Apo-Sul•fa•meth•ox•a•zole

Apo-Sul•fa•trim

Apo-Tet•ra

Apo-Tol•bu•ta•mide

Apo-Tri•mip

ap•pa•rat•us *pl.* ap•pa•rat•us, ap•pa•rat•us•es
biliary a.
digestive a.
a. digestorius
von Petz suturing a.
Wangensteen's a.
Wangensteen suction a.

ap•pear•ance
beaklike a.

ap•pear•ance *(continued)*
bull's-eye a.
cloverleaf a.
cobblestone a.
coiled-spring a.
corkscrew a.
ground-glass a.
lead pipe a.
mushroom and stem a.
pinwheel a.
pseudo–Billroth I a.
pseudotumor a.
sausagelike a.
sawtoothed a.
soap-sudsy a.
spiculated a.
stacked-coin a.
target a.
through-and-through a.
wind-sock a.

ap•pen•dage
cecal a.
epiploic a's
fibrous a. of liver
vermicular a.

ap•pen•da•gi•tis
epiploic a.

ap•pen•dec•to•my
incidental a.

ap•pen•di•cec•to•my

ap•pen•di•ci•tis
actinomycotic a.
acute a.
amebic a.
chronic a.
a. by contiguity
foreign-body a.
fulminating a.
gangrenous a.
helminthic a.
left-sided a.
lumbar a.
a. obliterans
obstructive a.
perforating a.

ap•pen•di•ci•tis *(continued)*
perforative a.
protective a.
purulent a.
recurrent a.
relapsing a.
segmental a.
skip a.
stercoral a.
subperitoneal a.
suppurative a.
traumatic a.
verminous a.

ap•pen•di•co•ce•cos•to•my

ap•pen•di•co•cele

ap•pen•di•co•en•ter•os•to•my

ap•pen•di•co•li•thi•a•sis

ap•pen•di•co•ly•sis

ap•pen•di•cop•a•thy

ap•pen•di•cos•to•my

ap•pen•dic•u•lar

ap•pen•dix *pl.* ap•pen•di•ces, ap•pen•dix•es
cecal a.
epiploic appendices
appendices epiploicae
a. fibrosa hepatis
fibrous a. of liver
inflamed a.
omental appendices
appendices omentales
a. vermicularis
vermiform a.
a. vermiformis

ap•pen•do•li•thi•a•sis

ap•pe•tite

ap•pli•ca•tor

ap•pli•er
cotton-tipped a.
endoclip a.

Ap•po•li•to
A's suture

ap•proach
Henry a.

APPY
appendectomy

APR
abdominal-perineal resection
abdominoperineal resection

aprin•dine

aproc•tia

apro•ti•nin

Aque•ous Char•co•dote

arab•i•no•side 5′-mono•phos•phate

ara-C
cytarabine

arach•i•don•ic ac•id

Aran•ti•us
A's ligament

ARC
AIDS-related complex

ar•cade
pancreatic a's
pancreatic a., anterior
pancreatic a., posterior

arch
tendinous a. of levator ani muscle

ar•cus *pl.* ar•cus
a. tendineus musculi levatoris ani

ARD
anorectal dressing

area *pl.* areae, areas
bare a. of liver
a. nuda hepatis

area *(continued)*
retroperitoneal a.
suprarenal a. of liver

ar•gi•nine

Ar•gyle In•gram tro•car cath•e•ter

ar•gy•ro•phil

A ring

Ar•i•zo•na

aro•ma•tase

Ar•res•tin

ar•te•ria *pl.* ar•te•riae
a. appendicularis
a. caecalis anterior
a. caecalis posterior
a. caudae pancreatis
a. colica dextra
a. colica media
a. colica sinistra
arteriae duodenales
a. epigastrica inferior
a. epigastrica superficialis
a. epigastrica superior
arteriae gastricae breves
a. gastrica dextra
a. gastrica posterior
a. gastrica sinistra
a. gastroduodenalis
a. gastroepiploica dextra
a. gastroepiploica sinistra
a. gastro-omentalis dextra
a. gastro-omentalis sinistra
a. hepatica communis
a. hepatica propria
arteriae ilei
a. ileocolica
arteriae intestinales
arteriae jejunales
a. lienalis
a. mesenterica inferior
a. mesenterica superior
a. pancreatica dorsalis
a. pancreatica inferior

ar•te•ria *(continued)*
 a. pancreatica magna
 arteriae pancreaticoduodenales inferiores
 a. pancreaticoduodenalis superior anterior
 a. pancreaticoduodenalis superior posterior
 a. rectalis inferior
 a. rectalis media
 a. rectalis superior
 arteriae sigmoideae
 a. splenica

ar•te•ri•og•ra•phy
 hepatic a.

ar•te•rio•scle•ro•sis
 gastric a.

ar•te•ry
 anterior cecal a.
 anterior superior pancreaticoduodenal a.
 appendicular a.
 ascending ileocolic a.
 caliber-persistent a. of the stomach
 caudal pancreatic a.
 colic a., left
 colic a., middle
 colic a., right
 cystic a.
 dorsal pancreatic a.
 a. of Drummond
 gastric a., left
 gastric a., posterior
 gastric a., right
 gastric a's, short
 gastroduodenal a.
 gastroepiploic a., left
 gastroepiploic a., right
 gastro-omental a., left
 gastro-omental a., right
 great pancreatic a.
 hemorrhoidal a., inferior
 hemorrhoidal a., middle
 hemorrhoidal a., superior

ar•te•ry *(continued)*
 hepatic a.
 hepatic a., common
 hepatic a., proper
 ileal a's
 ileocolic a.
 jejunal a's
 lienal a.
 marginal a. (of Drummond)
 mesenteric a.
 mesenteric a., inferior
 mesenteric a., superior
 pancreatic a., great
 pancreatic a., inferior
 pancreatica magna a.
 pancreaticoduodenal a's, inferior
 pancreaticoduodenal a., posterior superior
 piriformis a.
 rectal a., inferior
 rectal a., middle
 rectal a., superior
 sigmoid a's
 splenic a.
 submucosal a.

AS
 anal sphincter

5-ASA
 mesalamine (5-acetylsalicylic acid)

Asa•col

as•ca•ri•a•sis

as•car•i•cid•al

as•car•i•cide

as•ca•rid

as•car•i•des

as•ca•ri•di•a•sis

as•ca•ri•do•sis

as•ca•ri•o•sis

As•ca•ris
A. lumbricoides

as•ca•ris *pl.* as•car•i•des

Asch•off
Rokitansky-A. ducts
Rokitansky-A. sinuses

as•ci•tes
cirrhotic a.
exudative a.
pancreatic a.

Asep•to sy•ringe

ASGE
American Society for Gastrointestinal Endoscopy

asi•a•lo•gly•co•pro•tein

ASLC
acute self-limited colitis

ASP
L -asparaginase

Asp
L -asparaginase

as•par•a•gin•ase
a.-*E. coli*
L -a.

as•par•a•gine

as•par•tate

as•par•tate ami•no•trans•fer•ase

A-Spas

ASPD
anterior superior pancreaticodudenal artery

as•pi•ra•tion
diagnostic a.
a. of gastric contents
Levin tube a.

as•pi•ra•tor
Thorek gallbladder a.

as•pi•rin
a., sodium bicarbonate, and citric acid

as•say
carcinoembryonic antigen (CEA) a.
erythrocyte lysis a.

as•sess•ment
nutritional a.

as•sis•tant
gastrointestinal a. (GIA)

Ast•ler-Col•ler
A-C. staging (for colorectal carcinoma)

As•tra•morph

AT
abdominal tympany

Ata•rax

ATF
ascitic tumor fluid

At•kin•son
Key-Med-A. endoprosthesis

at•o•ny
gastric a.

ATP
adenosine triphosphate

atre•sia
anal a.
a. ani
bile duct a.
biliary a.
duodenal a.
esophageal a.
extrahepatic bile duct a.
intestinal a.
prepyloric a.

atre•to•gas•tria

atre•to•sto•mia

at•ro•phy
acute yellow a.
crypt a.
gastric a.
healed yellow a.
intestinal a.
subacute a. of liver
subchronic a. of liver
Sudeck's a.
villous a.
yellow a.

at•ro•pine
difenoxin and a.
diphenoxylate and a.
a., hyoscyamine, scopolamine, and phenobarbital
a. and phenobarbital

At•tain tube feed•ing for•mu•la

at•ta•pul•gite

Au•er•bach
A's plexus

Aug•men•tin

Ault
A. intestinal occlusion clamp

au•to•cho•le•cys•tec•to•my

au•to•di•ges•tion

au•to•la•vage

au•to•plas•ty
peritoneal a.

ave•no•lith

Av•i•tene

AW
actual weight

Ax•id

ax•is *pl.* ax•es
celiac a.

Azac•tam

5-aza•cy•ti•dine

aza•thio•prine

Az•lin

az•lo•cil•lin

AZQ
aziridinybenzoquinone

az•tre•o•nam

Azul•fi•dine

BA
  bile acid
  biliary atresia

Bab•cock
  B. clamp
  B. forceps
  B. gallbladder retractor
  B. intestinal forceps
  B. technique
  Lahey-B. forceps

ba•cam•pi•cil•lin

ba•cille
  b. Calmette-Guérin (BCG)

Ba•cil•lus
  B. cereus

ba•cil•lus *pl.* ba•cil•li
  Calmette-Guérin b.
  dysentery bacilli
  Schmitz's b.
  Shiga b.
  Sonne-Duval b.
  Stanley b.

bac•i•tra•cin
  b. zinc

back•cut

back-dif•fu•sion
  hydrogen ion b.-d.

back•flow

Back•haus
  B. dilator
  B. towel clamp

Ba•con
  B. anoscope

bac•te•ri•um *pl.* bac•te•ria
  coliform b.
  colonic b.
  gram-negative b.
  gram-positive b.

bac•te•ri•um *(continued)*
  pathogenic b.

Bac•te•roi•da•ceae

Bac•te•roi•des
  B. fragilis
  B. melaninogenicus

Bac•to•cill

Bac•trim

bag
  Acme One Time enteral feeding b.
  coloplast b.
  colostomy b.
  Davol feeding b.
  Dobhoff enteral feeding b.
  Entri-Pak enteral feeding b.
  ileostomy b.
  Keofeed enteral feeding b.
  McGaw/Nutripro enteral feeding b.
  Perry b.
  Polar enteral feeding b.
  1090 Gavage B.
  Top-Fill enteral feeding b.
  Whitmore b.

Bain•bridge
  B. intestinal clamp
  B. intestinal forceps

Bakes
  B. dilator
  B. probe

bal•an•ti•di•a•sis

bal•an•tid•i•o•sis

Bal•an•tid•i•um
  B. coli

Bal•four
  B. retractor
  B. self-retaining retractor

Bal•four *(continued)*
B. technique

Ball
B. procedure
B's valves

ball
food b.

Bal•li
B. contraction

bal•loon
air-filled b.
fluid-filled b.
Fogarty b.
Grüntzig b.
latex b.
Sengstaken b.

bal•sal•a•zide

Bal•ser
B's fatty necrosis

band
anterior b. of colon
b's of colon, longitudinal
free b. of colon
Harris' b.
Ladd's b's
Lane's b's
mesocolic b.
omental b.
retention b.

band•ing
suction b.

Ban•thine

BAO
basal acid output

Bar•bi•don•na

Bar•bi•don•na No. 2

Bar•bi•ta

Bard
B.-Parker blade
B.-Parker knife

bar•i•um
air-contrast b. enema
b. enema
nonflocculating b.
b. sulfate

Barnes
B. common duct dilator

Bar•o•phen

Baro•sperse

Barr
B. fistula hook
B. fistula probe

Bar•rett
B's epithelium
B's esophagus
B. intestinal forceps
B's syndrome
B's ulcer
B.-Clagett esophagogastrostomy
B.-Murphy intestinal thumb forceps

bar•ri•er
gastric mucosal b.

Bar•ron
B. ligation
B. Ligator

Barth
B's hernia

ba•sal

Ba•sal•jel

bas•cule
cecal b.

bas•ket
Dormia b.
Glassman b.
retrieval b.
sphincterotomy b.
spiral b.
stone extraction b.
trapped b.

ba•so•lat•er•al

Bas•sen
B.-Kornzweig disease

Bas•si•ni
B's operation

bath
sitz b.

Bat•tle
B. incision
B's operation
B.-Jalaguier-Kammerer incision

Bau•hin
B's valve

Baum•gar•ten
Cruveilhier-B. cirrhosis
Cruveilhier-B. syndrome

B bile

BC
biliary colic

BCAA
branched chain amino acid

BCNU
carmustine

BCO
biliary cholesterol output

BDL
bile duct ligation

BE
barium enema
Barrett's esophagus

Beal
Longmire and Beal gastric reservoir

Beards•ley
B. cecostomy trocar
B. intestinal clamp
B. intestinal forceps

Bearn
B.-Kunkel syndrome

Bearn *(continued)*
B.-Kunkel-Slater syndrome

Bea•ver
B. dissector

Beck
B. abdominal scoop
B. aorta forceps
B. gastrostomy
B.-Jianu gastrostomy
Kapp-B. colon clamp

Bé•clard
B's hernia

bec•lo•meth•a•sone

Beebe
B. hemostatic forceps

Beh•çet
B's syndrome

belch•ing

Bel•la•de•nal

bel•la•don•na
b. and butabarbital
kaolin, pectin, b. alkaloids, and opium
b. and phenobarbital

Bel•la•fo•line

Bell•al•phen

Bell/ans

Bel•lis
B. herniorrhaphy
Usher-B. hernia repair

bel•ly
wooden b.

Bel•sey
B. Mark IV operation

Ben•e•dict
B. gastroscope

ben•ox•a•pro•fen

Ben•son
B. pylorus separator

Ben•tyl

Ben•ty•lol

Ben•za•cot

ben•zal•de•hyde

ben•zal•de•hyde-de•hy•dro•gen•ase

ben•zo•di•az•e•pine

ben•zyl chlo•ride

Ber•ko•witz
B.-Bellis herniorrhaphy

Ber•nard
B's duct
B's glandular layer

Bern•stein
B. test

Best
B. colon clamp

Be•sure tube feed•ing for•mu•la

be•ta•meth•a•sone
b. sodium phosphate

be•thane•chol

Beth•a•prim

Be•thune
B. shears

BEV
bleeding esophageal varices

Bev•an
B. gallbladder forceps
B's incision

be•zoar
orange b.

BF
bile flow

BG
basic gastrin
bicolor guaiac

BICAP he•mo•stat•ic sys•tem

BICAP probe

bi•car•bo•nate

BiCNU

Bi•fi•do•bac•te•ri•um

BIL
bilirubin

Bil•a•gog

Bil•ax

Bil•boa
B.-Dotter tube

bile
A b.
b. acid
B b.
C b.
canalicular b.
cystic b.
extravasated b.
gallbladder b.
hepatic b.
inspissated b.
limy b.
milk of calcium b.
b. salt
white b.

bile ac•id
primary b.a.
secondary b.a.
tertiary b.a.

bile salt–stim•u•lat•ed lip•ase (BSSL)

bili.
bilirubin

bil•i•a•ry

bil•i•a•tion

bil•i•cy•a•nin

bil•i•fla•vin

bil•i•ful•vin

bil•i•fus•cin

bil•i•gen•e•sis

bil•i•ge•net•ic

bil•i•gen•ic

bil•i•hu•min

bi•lin

bil•ious

bil•i•pra•sin

bil•i•ru•bin
    b. conjugate
    conjugated b.
    direct b.
    direct-reacting b.
    b. ester conjugate
    b. glucuronide
    indirect b.
    indirect-reacting b.
    b. protein conjugate
    serum b.
    unconjugated b.
    urine b.

bil•i•ru•bi•nate

bil•i•ru•bin•ic

bil•i•ru•bi•nom•e•ter
    direct-reading b.

bil•i•ru•bino•sta•sis

bil•i•ver•din

bil•i•ver•din re•duc•tase

Bili•vist

bil•i•xan•thin

bil•i•xan•thine

Bill•roth
    B. hypertrophy
    B's operation
    Schoemaker-B. II
      technique

bi•lo•ma

Bil•opaque

bi•op•sy
    aspiration b.
    blind b.
    colonic b.
    duodenal b.
    esophageal b.
    fine-needle b.
    fine-needle aspiration b.
    hot b.
    intestinal b.
    jejunal drainage and b.
    large-forceps b.
    large-particle b.
    liver b.
    mucosal b.
    percutaneous liver b.
    peroral jejunal b.
    rectal b.
    scan-directed b.
    snare-excision b.
    transcutaneous b.
    transpapillary b.
    transvenous liver b.

Bio•search 7000 en•ter•al
  feed•ing pump

Bio•search 7005 en•ter•al
  feed•ing pump

bio•syn•the•sis

bio•tin

Birt•cher
    B. procto-sigmoid
      desiccation set

Bi•sac-Evac

bis•ac•o•dyl
    b. and docusate

Bi•sa•co•lax

bis•an•trene

Bis•co-Lax

bis•muth
b. subnitrate
b. subsalicylate

Bis•o•dol

bi•thi•o•nol

Black-Draught

Black-Draught Lax-Sen•na

blad•der
gall b.

blade
Bard-Parker b.

Blake
Ratliff-B. gallstone forceps

Blake•more
Sengstaken-B. tube

Bla•lock
B. pulmonary artery forceps

Blan•chard
B. hemorrhoid forceps

Blas•to•cys•tis
B. hominis

bleed
acute b.
GI (gastrointestinal) b.
UGI (upper gastrointestinal) b.

bleed•er

bleed•ing
diverticular b.
gastrointestinal (GI) b.
intestinal b.
lower gastrointestinal b.
mucosal b.
rectal b.
upper gastrointestinal b.
variceal b.

BLEO
bleomycin sulfate

Bleo
bleomycin sulfate

ble•o•my•cin
b. sulfate

blind•gut

bloat•ing

block•age
stoma b.

block•er
beta-adrenergic b.
calcium channel b.
H2 (histamine) b.

blood
bright red b.
bright red b. per rectum
occult b.

Blood•good
B. procedure

BLQ
both lower quadrants

BLS
blind loop syndrome

blue
brilliant b., C.
carmine b.
Evans b.
methylene b.
toluidine b.

Blum•berg
B's sign
inguinal ligament of B.

BM
basal metabolism

BMR
basal metabolic rate
basal metabolism rate

BNO
bowels not open

BO
bowel

BO *(continued)*
bowel obstruction
bowels open

Bo•as
B. point

Bo•den•heim•er
B. anoscope

body
acidophilic b.
cyanobacteria-like b.
foreign b.
b. of gallbladder
gastric b.
Jaworski b's
ketone b's
Leishman-Donovan b.
Mallory's b's
Nothnagel's b's
b. of stomach
vermiform b's

Boeck
B's sarcoma

Boehm
B. anoscope
B. proctoscope
B. rectal diagnostic and treatment set
B. sigmoidoscope

Boer•haave
B's syndrome

Boldt
Mayo-B. appendix inverter

bol•ster
rubber b.

bo•lus
alimentary b.

bom•be•sin

Bon•nell
B. suture

Bon•ney
B. dissecting forceps

BOR
bowels open regularly

bor•bo•ryg•mus *pl.* bor•bo•ryg•mi

bor•rel•i•o•sis
B. classification (for advanced gastric cancer)

Bou•chard
B's disease

bou•gie
Hurst's b's
Klebanoff common duct b.
Maloney b.
mercury-filled b.
Savary b.
Wales rectal b.

Bo•vie
B. electrosurgical unit

bow•el
decompression of b.
defunctionalized b.
b. prep
proximal b.

Boyce
B's sign

Boy•den
B. test meal
sphincter of B.

Boze•man
B. forceps

Bo•zi•ce•vich
B's test

BPC
bile phospholipid concentration

BPO
bile phospholipid output

BPR
blood per rectum

BPRS
  brief psychiatric reacting scale

BR
  bowel rest

brachy•esoph•a•gus

Brad•ley
  B's disease

brady•ki•nin

brake
  duodenal b.
  ileal b.

brash
  water b.

BRAT
  bananas, rice cereal, applesauce, tea (diet)

Braun
  B's anastomosis
  B. and Jaboulay technique

BRB
  bright red blood

BRBPR
  bright red blood per rectum

breath
  liver b.

bre•fel•din

BRIC
  benign recurrent intrahepatic cholestasis

Bridge
  B. deep surgery forceps

bri•dle
  feeding tube b.

B ring

Brin•ker•hoff
  B. anoscope
  B. rectal speculum

Brin•ker•hoff *(continued)*
  B's speculum

Brin•ton
  B's disease

Broe•sike
  B's fossa

bro•mo•ben•zene

Bro•mo-Selt•zer

Brom•sul•pha•lein

Brooke
  B. ileostomy

Brooks
  B. gallbladder scissors

Brown
  Adson-B. forceps
  B's method
  B. needle holder

bru•cel•lo•sis

Brun•ner
  B's glands
  B's gland adenoma
  B's gland hyperplasia
  B. intestinal forceps
  B. ligature set
  B. tissue forceps

Brun•schwig
  B's operation

brush
  cleaning b.
  cytology b.
  endoscopic b.
  Glassman b.
  sheathed cytology b.
  stomach b.

BS
  bile salt

BSA
  bowel sounds active

BSC
  bile salt concentration

BSD
baby soft diet
bedside drainage

BSM
bile salt metabolism

BSN
bowel sounds normal

BSNA
bowel sounds normal and active

BSO
bile salt output

BSR
bowel sounds regular

BSS
balanced salt solution
black silk suture

BSSL
bile salt–stimulated lipase

BT
bowel tones

BTP
biliary tract pain

BTP (*N*-benzoyl-L-tyrosyl-*p*-aminobenzoic acid) test

bub•ble
air b.

bu•bono•cele

bu•cry•late

Budd
B.-Chiari disease
B.-Chiari syndrome

bu•de•son•ide

Buie
B. biopsy forceps
B. fistula probe
B. fulguration electrode
B. pile clamp
B. position
B. rectal injection cannula

Buie *(continued)*
B. rectal operating scissors
B. rectal suction tip
B. sigmoidoscope
B.-Hirschman anoscope
B.-Smith anal retractor
Smith-B. anal retractor

bulb
duodenal b.

bu•lim•ia

bulk
tumor b.

bulk•age

BUN
blood urea nitrogen

bu•piv•a•caine

bu•pre•nor•phine

BUQ
both upper quadrants

Bu•row
B's vein

bur•sa *pl.* bur•sae
omental b.
b. omentalis

bur•si•tis
omental b.

Busch
B. umbilical scissors

Bu•sco•pan

Bu•si
B. contraction

Bu•so•di•um

bu•ta•bar•bi•tal
belladonna and b.

Bu•tal•an

Bu•ti•bel

Bu•ti•sol

but•ton
- gastrostomy feeding b.
- Jaboulay b.
- Murphy's b.
- peritoneal b.

bu•ty•rate

BW
- body weight

By•clo•mine

By•ler
- B's disease

by•pass
- colonic b.
- gastric b.
- intestinal b.
- jejunal b.
- jejunoileal b.
- partial ileal b.

C

CA 50 (tumor marker)

CA 19-9 (tumor marker)

CA 195 (tumor marker)

Ca-ATPase
  calcium-ATPase

ca•chec•tin

ca•chex•ia

cad•mi•um

cae•cum

cae•cus
  c. minor ventriculi

CAG
  cholangiogram
  chronic atrophic gastritis

CAH
  chronic active hepatitis

cake
  omental c.

cal•bin•din
  subserosal c.

Cal•ci•lac

cal•ci•to•nin

cal•ci•um
  alumina, magnesia, and c. carbonate
  biliary c.
  c. carbonate
  c. carbonate and magnesia
  c. carbonate, magnesia, and simethicone
  c. carbonate and simethicone
  c. glubionate
  ionized serum c.
  c. and magnesium carbonates
  c. polycarbophil

cal•ci•um *(continued)*
  simethicone, alumina, c. carbonate, and magnesia

cal•ci•um aden•o•sine•tri•phos•pha•tase

cal•ci•um-ATP•ase

cal•cu•lus *pl.* cal•cu•li
  alvine c.
  gastric c.
  hepatic c.
  intestinal c.
  pancreatic c.
  shellac c.
  stomachic c.

CALD
  chronic active liver disease

Cal•gly•cine

cal•i•ci•vi•rus

cal•mod•u•lin

cal•o•rim•e•try
  indirect c.

Ca•lot
  C's triangle

Cal Pow•der cal•o•rie sup•ple•ment

cal•pro•tec•tin

cal•ret•i•nin

CAM-1189

Cam•a•lox

cam•era
  endoscopic still c.

Cam•er•on
  C. electrosurgical unit
  C. flexible gastroscope
  C.-Miller electrocoagulation unit

Cam•er•on *(continued)*
C.-Miller monopolar electrode
C.-Miller suction-coagulator

Cam•il•leri
C. classification (for vascular anomalies of the gastrointestinal tract)

cam•o•stat

cAMP
cyclic adenosine monophosphate

Cam•per
C's fascia
fascia of C.

camp•to•the•cin

Cam•py•lo•bac•ter
C. coli
C. fetus subsp. *fetus*
C. jejuni

Can•a•da
Cronkhite-C. polyp
Cronkhite-C. syndrome

ca•nal
alimentary c.
anal c.
biliary c's, interlobular
biliary c's, intralobular
digestive c.
gastric c.
c's of Hering
hernial c.
intestinal c.
c. of Nuck
portal c.
pyloric c.
Santorini's c.
c. of stomach
ventricular c.
c. of Wirsung

can•a•lic•u•lus *pl.* can•a•lic•u•li

can•a•lic•u•lus *(continued)*
bile canaliculi
biliary canaliculi
intracellular canaliculi of parietal cells
pseudobile c.

ca•na•lis *pl.* ca•na•les
c. alimentarius
c. analis
c. gastricus
c. pyloricus
c. ventricularis
c. ventriculi

can•cer
anal c.
biliary tract c.
colon c.
colonic c.
colorectal c.
disseminated c.
duodenal c.
endocrine c.
esophageal c.
esophagogastric junction c.
familial colon c.
gallbladder c.
gastric c.
GI c.
hereditary nonpolyposis colon c.
hereditary nonpolyposis colorectal c.
intestinal c.
large bowel c.
liver c.
nonfixed c.
obstructing c.
pancreatic c.
periampullary c.
resectable c.
small intestinal c.
synchronous c.

Can•di•da
C. albicans

can•nu•la
blunt c.

can•nu•la *(continued)*
Buie rectal injection c.
Cremer c.
Franklin-Silverman biopsy c.
Ingalls rectal injection c.
Medicut c.
Teflon ERCP c.

can•nu•la•tion

Can•til

Can•tor
C. tube

ca. ox.
calcium oxalate

CAP
chronic alcoholic pancreatitis

cap
bishop's c.
duodenal c.
phrygian c.
pyloric c.

ca•pac•i•ty
serum iron-binding c.

Cap•il•lar•ia
C. philippinensis

cap•il•la•ri•a•sis
hepatic c.

cap•il•lar•itis

cap•il•lary
bile c's
submucosal c.

ca•pote•ment

cap•su•la *pl.* cap•su•lae
c. fibrosa [Glissoni] c.
c. fibrosa hepatis
c. fibrosa perivascularis
c. pancreatis

cap•sule
biopsy c.
Crosby c.

cap•sule *(continued)*
fibrous c. of liver
Glisson's c.
hepatobiliary c.
c. of pancreas
radiotelemetering c.
telemetering c.

cap•su•li•tis
hepatic c.

cap•to•pril

cap•ut *pl.* cap•i•ta
c. pancreatis

Car•a•fate

CARB
carbohydrate

car•ba•chol

car•ba•maz•e•pine

car•ben•i•cil•lin

car•bo•hy•drate
dietary c.

car•bon
c. tetrachloride

car•bo•pla•tin

car•box•yl•ic es•ter hy•dro•lase

car•boxy•meth•yl•cel•lu•lose
psyllium hydrophilic mucilloid and c.

car•boxy•pep•ti•dase

car•boxy•pep•ti•dase A

car•boxy•pep•ti•dase B

car•ci•no•em•bry•on•ic

car•cin•o•gen
genotoxic c.

car•ci•no•gen•e•sis

car•ci•noid
gastric c.

car•ci•no•ma *pl.* car•ci•no•mas, car•ci•no•ma•ta
acinar hepatocellular c.
cholangiocellular c.
clear cell hepatocellular c.
diffuse hepatocellular c.
fibrolamellar hepatocellular c.
hepatocellular c.
hepatocellular c., acinar
hepatocellular c., clear cell
hepatocellular c., diffuse
hepatocellular c., fibrolamellar
hepatocellular c., scirrhous
hepatocellular c., solid
hepatocellular c., trabecular
hepatocellular c., undifferentiated
hereditary nonpolyposis colorectal c.
c. in situ
intramucosal c.
invasive c.
mixed hepatocellular c.–cholangiocarcinoma
mucoepidermoid c.
squamous c.

car•ci•no•sar•co•ma

car•dia

car•di•ac

car•di•ec•to•my

Car•di•llo
C. retractor

car•dio•esoph•a•ge•al

car•dio•my•ot•o•my

car•dio•plas•ty

car•dio•py•lo•ric

car•dio•spasm

car•di•ot•o•my

Ca•rey
Coons/C. endoprosthesis

Car•man
C.-Kirklin meniscus complex
C.-Kirklin meniscus sign

Car•mel
C. clamp

car•mine
indigo c.

car•mus•tine

car•ni•tine

Car•oid Lax•a•tive

Ca•ro•li
C's disease

car•ri•er
ligature c.

car•un•cle
major c. of Santorini

ca•san•thra•nol
c. and docusate

cas•cara
mineral oil and c. sagrada
c. sagrada and aloe
c. sagrada and phenolphthalein

Ca•sec pro•tein mod•ule

ca•sein

Case Pow•der pro•tein sup•ple•ment

cast
hair c.

cas•tor oil

CAT
computed abdominal tomography

cat•e•chol•amine

CATH
  catheter

ca•thar•tic

ca•thep•sin

cath•e•ter
  Argyle Ingram trocar c.
  balloon c.
  blunt c.
  cannulating c.
  cecostomy c.
  central venous c.
  Cobra c.
  drainage c.
  Eisenberg c.
  Fogarty c.
  Foley bag c.
  Foley c.
  Formacath c.
  Gruentzig c.
  guide c.
  headhunter c.
  indwelling c.
  Lane gastroenterostomy c.
  Malecot c.
  Medicut c.
  Medi-Tech steerable c.
  microtip transducer c.
  mushroom c.
  mushroom-tip c.
  nasobiliary c.
  oral c.
  Pezzer's c.
  pigtail c.
  polyethylene c.
  polyvinylchloride (PVC) c.
  PTHC c.
  Ring c.
  Robinson c.
  SIM 2 c.
  Simmons c.
  Teflon c.
  toposcopic c.
  transanal c.
  transducer c.
  water-perfused c.

cath•e•ter•iza•tion
  transhepatic c.

CATS
  combined abdominal transsacral resection technique

Cat•tell
  C. T-tube

cau•da *pl.* cau•dae
  c. pancreatis

caul

cau•tery
  endoscopic c.

cav•i•tas *pl.* cav•i•ta•tes
  c. peritonealis

cav•i•ty
  peritoneal c.
  peritoneal c., greater
  peritoneal c., lesser

CB
  conjugated bilirubin

CBD
  common bile duct

CBDE
  common bile duct exploration

CBH
  chronic benign hepatitis

C bile

CCD (charge-coupled device) en•do•scope

CCK
  cholecystokinin

CCK-LI
  cholecystokinin-like immunoreactivity

CCK-OP
  cholecystokinin octapeptide

CCL 277 (colon cancer) cells

CCNU
  lomustine

CCS
  cholecystosonography
  Cronkhite-Canada syndrome

CD
  Crohn's disease

CDAI
  Crohn's Disease Activity Index

CE
  cardioesophageal
  cholesteryl esters

CEA
  carcinoembryonic antigen

ce•ca

ce•cal

ce•cec•to•my

ce•ci•tis

ce•co•cele

ce•co•col•ic

ce•co•co•lon

ce•co•co•lo•pexy

ce•co•co•los•to•my

ce•co•fix•a•tion

ce•co•il•e•ost•o•my

ce•co•pexy

ce•co•pli•ca•tion

ce•cor•rha•phy

ce•co•sig•moid•os•to•my

ce•cos•to•my
  "blow-hole" c.

ce•cot•o•my

ce•cum
  coned c.
  high c.
  c. mobile
  mobile c.

CeeNU

ce•fix•ime

Ce•fi•zox

cef•met•a•zole

Cef•o•bid

cef•o•per•a•zone

Cef•o•tan

cef•o•tax•ime

cef•o•te•tan

ce•fox•i•tin

cef•ta•zi•dime

cef•ti•zox•ime

cef•tri•a•xone

CEH
  carboxylic ester hydrolase

Ce•les•tin
  Medoc-C. endoprosthesis

Ce•les•tone

ce•li•ac

ce•li•ec•to•my

ce•lio•en•ter•ot•o•my

ce•lio•gas•trot•o•my

ce•lio•scope

ce•li•os•co•py

ce•li•ot•o•my
  ventral c.

cell
  absorptive c.
  absorptive c., intestinal
  acid c.
  acinar c.

cell *(continued)*
acinous c.
algoid c's
argyrophil c.
border c's
CaCo2 c.
caveolated c's
central c.
centroacinar c's
chief c's
COLO 320 (colon cancer) c.
D c's
Davidoff's c's
dendritic c's
ECL (argyrophil) c.
endothelial c.
enterochromaffin-like c.
epithelial c's
fat-storing c's of liver
gastrin c.
goblet c.
H-35 (hepatoma) c.
Heidenhain's c's
hepatic c's
hepG2 (Hepatoma) c.
HLF (hepatoma) c.
HT-29 (colon cancer) c.
IEC-6 (intestinal epithelial) c.
interstitial c's
intestinal endocrine c.
IPEC-J2 (intestinal epithelial) c.
islet c's
JR-E (gastric cancer) c.
JR-St (gastric cancer) c.
KATO-III (gastric cancer) c.
Kupffer's c's
LIM 2537 (colon cancer) c.
liver c's
LLC-PK1 (renal cell carcinoma) c.
lymphokine-activated killer (LAK) c.
M c.
mast c.

cell *(continued)*
c. migration
mucous c's
mucous neck c's
multinucleated giant c.
natural killer c.
neuroendocrine c.
oxyntic c's
Paneth's c's
parietal c's
peptic c's
perisinusoidal c.
pit c.
PLC-PRF 5 (hepatoma) c.
secretory c.
SW 480 (colon cancer) c.
T84 (colon cancer) c.
^{99m}Tc-labeled red blood c's
technetium 99m–labeled red blood c's
villus c.
von Kupffer's c's
zymogenic c's

Cel•len
C's sign

celo•scope

ce•los•co•py

ce•lot•o•my

Ceo-Two

ceph•a•lo•cyst

cer•am•i•dase

cer•car•ia *pl.* cer•car•iae

cer•car•i•ci•dal

ce•ru•lo•plas•min

Ces•to•da

ces•tode

ces•to•di•a•sis

Cey•lon sore mouth

CGRP
calcitonin gene–related peptide

Ch
cholesterol

CHA
common hepatic artery

Chaf•fin
C. sump tube

Cha•gas
C. disease

chal•lenge
gluten c.
jejunal gluten c.
rectal gluten c.

Cham•ber•lin
Eder-C. gastroscope

chan•nel
calcium c.
chloride c.
ion c.
suction c.

Char•co•aid

char•coal
activated c.

Char•co•caps

Char•cot
C's fever
C's syndrome
C's triad

Char•don•na-2

Chas•sard
C.-Lapiné projection

Chauf•fard
C's point

Chea•tle
C.-Henry incision

chel•o•sol

Chel•sea
C.-Eaton anal speculum

che•mo•dis•so•lu•tion

che•mo•tax•is

che•mo•ther•a•py
adjuvant c.
intra-arterial c.

Che•nix

che•no•de•oxy•cho•late

che•no•de•oxy•cho•lic acid

che•no•di•ol

che•no•ther•a•py

Cher•a•gan W/TMP

Cher•nez
C. incision

Che•va•li•er
C. gastroscope

Chi•a•ri
Budd-C. disease
Budd-C. syndrome
C's disease
C's syndrome

Chi•ba
C. needle

Chi•lai•di•ti
C. syndrome

Child
C's classification
C. intestinal forceps
C. operation

Chil•dren's Hos•pi•tal in•tes•ti•nal for•ceps

Childs
C.-Phillips intestinal plication needle

Chi•lo•mas•tix

CHL
chlorambucil

Chl
  chlorambucil

Chla•myd•ia
  C. trachomatis

chla•myd•ia *pl.* chla•myd•iae

chla•myd•i•al

chlor•am•bu•cil

chlor•am•phen•i•col

chlor•de•cone

chlor•di•az•ep•ox•ide
  c. and clidinium

chlor•et•ic

chlor•hy•dria

chlo•ride

chlor•id•or•rhea
  familial c.

Chlo•ro•my•ce•tin

chlo•ro•quine

chlo•ro•zo•to•cin

chlor•prom•a•zine

chlor•zox•a•zone

CHOL
  cholesterol

Cho•lac

chol•a•gog•ic

chol•a•gogue

cho•lan•e•re•sis

cho•lan•ge•itis

cho•lan•gi•ec•ta•sis

cho•lan•gio•car•ci•no•ma
  hilar c.
  mixed hepatocellular carcinoma–c.
  peripheral c.

cho•lan•gio•cho•le•cys•to•cho•le•doch•ec•tomy

cho•lan•gio•en•ter•os•to•my

cho•lan•gio•gas•tros•to•my

cho•lan•gio•gram
  catheter c.
  fine-needle c.
  T-tube c.

cho•lan•gi•og•ra•phy
  fine needle transhepatic c. (FNTC)
  operative c.
  percutaneous transhepatic c. (PTHC)
  T-tube c.

cho•lan•gio•hep•a•ti•tis

cho•lan•gio•je•ju•nos•to•my
  intrahepatic c.

cho•lan•gi•o•lar

cho•lan•gi•ole

cho•lan•gi•o•li•tis

chol•an•gio•pan•cre•a•tos•co•py
  peroral c. (PCPS)

chol•an•gio•scope

chol•an•gi•os•co•py
  peroral c.

cho•lan•gi•os•to•my

cho•lan•gi•ot•o•my

cho•lan•gio•ve•nous

cho•lan•gi•tis
  acute obstructive suppurative c.
  ascending c.
  bacterial c.
  chronic nonsuppurative destructive c.
  c. lenta
  obstructive c.
  posttransplantation c.
  primary sclerosing c.

cho·lan·gi·tis *(continued)*
progressive
nonsuppurative c.
rejection c.
sclerosing c.
suppurative c.

Cho·lan-HMB

cho·lano·poi·e·sis

cho·lano·poi·et·ic

cho·late

cho·le·bil·i·ru·bin

Cho·le·brine

cho·le·chro·mo·poi·e·sis

cho·le·cy·a·nin

cho·le·cyst

cholecyst.
cholecystectomy

cho·le·cyst·a·gog·ic

cho·le·cyst·a·gogue

cho·le·cys·tat·o·ny

cho·le·cys·tec·ta·sia

cho·le·cys·tec·to·my
laparoscopic c.

cho·le·cys·ten·ter·ic

cho·le·cyst·en·tero·anas·to·mo·sis

cho·le·cyst·en·ter·or·rha·phy

cho·le·cyst·en·ter·os·to·my

cho·le·cyst·gas·tros·to·my

cho·le·cys·tic

cho·le·cys·tis

cho·le·cys·ti·tis
acalculous c.
acute c.
chronic c.

cho·le·cys·ti·tis *(continued)*
c. emphysematosa
emphysematous c.
follicular c.
gaseous c.
c. glandularis proliferans

cho·le·cyst·ne·phros·to·my

cho·le·cys·to·co·lon·ic

cho·le·cys·to·co·los·to·my

cho·le·cys·to·co·lot·o·my

cho·le·cys·to·du·o·de·nal

cho·le·cys·to·du·o·de·nos·to·my

cho·le·cys·to·en·ter·os·to·my

cho·le·cys·to·gas·tric

cho·le·cys·to·gas·tros·to·my

cho·le·cys·to·gog·ic
oral c.

cho·le·cys·to·il·e·os·to·my

cho·le·cys·to·in·tes·ti·nal

cho·le·cys·to·je·ju·nos·to·my

cho·le·cys·to·ki·net·ic

cho·le·cys·to·ki·nin
c. octapeptide (CCK-OP)

cho·le·cys·to·li·thi·a·sis

cho·le·cys·to·litho·trip·sy

cho·le·cys·to·ne·phros·to·my

cho·le·cys·top·a·thy

cho·le·cys·to·pexy

cho·le·cys·top·to·sis

cho·le·cys·to·py·elos·to·my

cho·le·cys·tor·rha·phy

cho•le•cys•tos•co•py
percutaneous transhepatic c.

cho•le•cys•to•sis
hyperplastic c.

cho•le•cys•tos•to•my

cho•le•cys•tot•o•my

cho•le•doch•al

cho•le•do•chec•to•my

cho•le•do•chen•dy•sis

cho•le•do•chi•tis

cho•led•o•cho•cele

cho•led•o•cho•chol•e•do•chos•to•my

cho•led•o•cho•du•o•de•nos•to•my

cho•led•o•cho•en•ter•os•to•my

cho•le•do•cho•fi•ber•scope

cho•led•o•cho•gas•tros•to•my

cho•led•o•cho•hep•a•tos•to•my

cho•led•o•cho•il•e•os•to•my

cho•led•o•cho•je•ju•nos•to•my

cho•led•o•cho•lith

cho•led•o•cho•li•thi•a•sis

cho•led•o•cho•li•thot•o•my

cho•led•o•cho•litho•trip•sy

cho•led•o•cho•plas•ty
percutaneous c.

cho•led•o•chor•rha•phy

cho•led•o•cho•scope
fiber c.

cho•led•o•chos•to•my

cho•led•o•chot•o•my

cho•led•o•chus

cho•le•dos•co•py
cystic duct c.
jejunostomy tract c.
T-tube tract c.

cho•le-en•ter•ic

cho•le-en•ter•os•to•my

cho•le•glo•bin

Cho•le•gra•fin

cho•le•ic

cho•le•ic ac•id

cho•le•lith

cholelith.
cholelithiasis

cho•le•li•thi•a•sis

cho•le•lith•ic

cho•le•li•thot•o•my

cho•le•litho•trip•sy

cho•le•li•thot•ri•ty

cho•lem•e•sis

cho•le•mia
familial c.
Gilbert c.

cho•le•mic

cho•le•peri•to•ne•um

cho•le•peri•to•ni•tis

cho•le•poi•e•sis

cho•le•poi•et•ic

cho•le•pra•sin

chol•era
c. morbus
pancreatic c.
summer c.

cho•ler•e•sis

cho•ler•et•ic

choles.
  cholesterol

Cho•les•ta•byl

cho•le•sta•sia

cho•le•sta•sis
  benign postoperative intrahepatic c.
  bile ductular c.
  extrahepatic c.
  intrahepatic c.
  neonatal c.
  Norwegian c.
  pericentral c.
  progressive intrahepatic c.
  recurrent c.

cho•le•stat•ic

cho•les•ter•ol
  biliary c.

cho•les•ter•ol•er•e•sis

cho•les•ter•ol-7α-hy•droxy•lase

cho•les•ter•ol•o•sis
  acalculous c.

cho•les•ter•yl
  c. esters

cho•les•ty•ra•mine

Cho•le•tec

cho•let•e•lin

cho•le•ther•a•py

cho•le•ver•din

cho•lic acid

cho•line

cho•line ac•e•tyl•trans•fer•ase

cholo•chrome

cholo•cy•a•nin

cholo•ge•net•ic

Cho•lo•gra•fin

cholo•lith

cholo•li•thi•a•sis

cholo•lith•ic

cholo•poi•e•sis

Cho•ly•bar

Chooz

chro•mar•gen•taf•fin

chro•ma•tog•ra•phy
  high-performance liquid c.

chro•ma•to•pec•tic

chro•ma•to•pex•is

Chro•mi•tope

chro•mi•um
  c. sesquioxide

chro•mo•gran•in
  c. A

chro•mo•pec•tic

chro•mo•pex•ic

chro•mo•pexy

chro•mos•co•py

Chron•u•lac

CHRS
  cerebrohepatorenal syndrome

Church
  C. deep surgery scissors

chyle

chy•lo•me•di•as•ti•num

chy•lo•mi•cron *pl.* chyl•lo•mi•crons, chy•lo•mi•cra

chy•lo•peri•to•ne•um

chy•lus

chy•mo•tryp•sin

CIA
congenital intestinal aganglionosis

CIBD
chronic inflammatory bowel disease

Ci•dex

cIEL
crypt intraepithelial lymphocyte

CIIP
chronic idiopathic intestinal pseudo-obstruction

ci•la•stat•in
imipenem and c.

Cil•li•um

CIM
cimetidine

ci•met•i•dine

CINE
chemotherapy-induced nausea and emesis

cine•def•e•cog•ra•phy

cine•ra•di•og•ra•phy

Cip•ro

cip•ro•flox•a•cin

cir•cuit
short c.

cir•cu•la•tion
enterohepatic c.
portal c.
portoumbilical c.

cir•cum•anal

cir•cum•in•tes•ti•nal

cir•rho•sis
acute juvenile c.
alcoholic c.
atrophic c.

cir•rho•sis *(continued)*
bacterial c.
biliary c.
calculus c.
cardiac c.
congestive c.
Cruveilhier-Baumgarten c.
decompensated c.
fatty c.
focal biliary c.
glabrous c.
Hanot's c.
hypertrophic c.
Laënnec's c.
c. of liver
macronodular c.
malarial c.
medionodular c.
metabolic c.
micromedionodular c.
micronodular c.
mixed c.
multilobular c.
periportal c.
pigment c.
pigmentary c.
pipe stem c.
portal c.
posthepatitic c.
postnecrotic c.
primary biliary c.
secondary biliary c.
stasis c.
c. of stomach
syphilitic c.
Todd's c.
toxic c.
unilobular c.
vascular c.

cir•rhot•ic

CIS
carcinoma in situ

cis•a•pride

cis•pla•tin

cit•ric acid
- acetaminophen, calcium carbonate, potassium and sodium bicarbonates, and c.a.
- acetaminophen, sodium bicarbonate, and c.a.
- aspirin, sodium bicarbonate, and c.a.

Cit•ro•bac•ter
- *C. amalonaticus*
- *C. freundii*
- *C. intermedius*

Cit•ro•car•bon•ate

Cit•ro•ma

Cit•ro-Mag

Cit•ro-Ne•sia

Cit•ro•tein tube feed•ing for•mu•la

Cit•ru•cel

CK
- cholecystokinin

Cla•do
- C's ligament

Cla•for•an

Cla•gett
- C. esophagogastrostomy
- C.-Barrett esophagogastrostomy
- Waugh and C. operation

clamp
- Abadie enterostomy c.
- Allen intestinal c.
- Allen-Kocher c.
- Allis c.
- anastomosis c.
- Ault intestinal occlusion c.
- Babcock c.
- Backhaus towel c.
- Bainbridge intestinal c.
- Beardsley intestinal c.
- Best colon c.

clamp *(continued)*
- Buie pile c.
- Carmel c.
- cecostomy c.
- Collins umbilical c.
- colon c.
- colostomy c.
- Cope's c.
- Crile's c.
- curved Mayo c.
- Dean-MacDonald gastric resection c.
- DeMartel c.
- DeMartel-Wolfson c.
- Dennis c.
- Dixon-Thomas-Smith colon c.
- Doyen's c.
- Edna towel c.
- Fehland right angle colon c.
- Fogarty Hydrogrip c.
- Foss anterior resection c.
- Furniss anastomosis c.
- Furniss-Clute duodenal c.
- Gant's c.
- Glassman non-crushing gastrointestinal c.
- Gomco umbilical c.
- Hayes anterior resection c.
- Hayes colon c.
- hemorrhoidal c.
- hemostatic c.
- Hunt colostomy c.
- Hurwitz intestinal c.
- intestinal c.
- Jarvis pile c.
- Kane umbilical c.
- Kapp-Beck colon c.
- Kelly c.
- Köcher c.
- Lane gastroenterostomy c.
- McCleery-Miller anastomosis c.
- McNealy-Glassman c.
- Madden intestinal c.
- Martel's c.
- Mayo c.

clamp *(continued)*
metal wing c.
Mikulicz's c.
Mixter c.
Moreno gastroenterostomy c.
mosquito c.
Moynihan c.
Myles hemorrhoidal c.
Ochsner c.
Payr c.
Payr gastrointestinal c.
Payr pylorus c.
Péan c.
pedicle c.
Pemberton sigmoid anastomosis c.
Pennington c.
Phillips rectal c.
Rankin c.
Rankin anastomosis c.
Rankin intestinal c.
right angle c.
Roosevelt gastroenterostomy c.
rubber-sheathed c.
rubber-shod c.
Satinsky c.
Schnidt c.
Singley intestinal ring c.
Stone intestinal c.
towel c.
von Petz c.
von Petz stomach c.
Wangensteen anastomosis c.
Watts locking c.
Wertheim pedicle c.
Zachary Cope-DeMartel colon c.

clamp hold•er
DeMartel-Wolfson c.h.

cla•rith•ro•my•cin

Clark
C. common duct dilator

clas•si•fi•ca•tion
Borrmann c. (for advanced gastric cancer)
Camilleri c. (for vascular anomalies of the gastrointestinal tract)
Child's c. (for liver disease)
Dukes' c. (for colorectal carcinoma)
Gautier c. (for extrahepatic bile duct atresia)
Kasai c. (for extrahepatic bile duct atresia)
Kasugai c. (for chonic pancreatitis)
Lewis c. (for vascular anomalies of the gastrointestinal tract)
Ludwig-Dickson-MacDonald c. (for primary biliary cirrhosis)
Moore c. (for vascular anomalies of the gastrointestinal tract)
Rappaport c. (for non-Hodgkin's lymphoma)

Clas•son
C. deep surgery scissors

cla•vu•lan•ate
amoxicillin and c.
ticarcillin and c.

Cla•vu•lin

clear•ance
Bromsulphalein c.
esophageal acid c.

cli•din•i•um
chlordiazepoxide and c.

clin•da•my•cin

Clin•dex

Clin•ox•ide

clip
Kifa skin c.
Michel c.
Naso-Tube c.
von Petz suture c.

Clip•ox•ide

CLO
Campylobacter-like organisms

clog•ging
tube c.

clo•nor•chi•a•sis

Clo•nor•chis si•nen•sis

Clo•pra

Clo•quet
C's hernia

Clos•trid•i•um
C. botulinum
C. difficile
C. perfringens
C. tetani

clos•trid•i•um *pl.* clos•trid•ia

clo•sure
stapled c.
Tom Jones c.
Witzel c.

clot
fundic c.
sentinel c.

clox•a•cil•lin so•di•um

Clox•a•pen

clus•ter
hemorrhoidal c.

Clute
Furniss-C. duodenal clamp

Cly•so•drast

c-*myc* on•co•gene

co•ag•u•la•tion
bipolar c.

co•ag•u•la•tion *(continued)*
coaptive c.
direct current c.
electrohydrothermal (EHT) c.
infrared c.

co•ag•u•la•tor
Cameron-Miller suction-c.

coat
external c. of esophagus
vascular c. of stomach
villous c. of small intestine

co•bal•a•min

co•bal•oph•i•lin

cob•ble•stone
c. mucosa

Co•bel•li
C's glands

Co•bra cath•e•ter

coc•cid•i•al

coc•cid•i•an

Coc•cid•i•oi•des

coc•cid•i•oi•do•my•co•sis

coc•cid•i•um *pl.* coc•cid•ia

co•deine

Co•lace

Co•lax

col•chi•cine

Cole
C. duodenal retractor
Huppert-C. test

co•lec•to•my
elective c.
segmental c.
subtotal c.
total c.
total abdominal c.

Co•les•tid

co•les•ti•pol

col•ic
appendicular c.
biliary c.
bilious c.
endemic c.
flatulent c.
gallstone c.
gastric c.
hepatic c.
infant c.
intestinal c.
pancreatic c.
stercoral c.
vermicular c.
verminous c.
wind c.
worm c.

col•i•ca

col•icky

co•lip•ase
pancreatic c.

co•lip•ase-de•pen•dent lip•ase

co•li•pli•ca•tion

co•li•punc•ture

co•lit•i•des

co•li•tis *pl.* co•lit•i•des
acute self-limited c.
amebic c.
antibiotic-associated c.
balantidial c.
cathartic c.
chronic ulcerative c.
collagenous c.
Crohn's c.
c. cystica profunda
c. cystica superficialis
cytomegalovirus (CMV) c.
diversion c.
drug-induced c.
eosinophilic c.
fulminant c.
granulomatous c.

co•li•tis *(continued)*
c. gravis
infectious c.
irradiation c.
ischemic c.
lymphocytic c.
microscopic c.
mucosal ulcerative c.
mucous c.
neutropenic c.
c. polyposa
pseudomembranous c.
radiation c.
regional c.
segmental c.
sexually transmitted c.
transmural c.
c. ulcerativa
ulcerative c.

col•la•gen

col•la•gen•ase

col•lag•e•nous

col•lar
ulcer c.

Col•lin
C. intestinal forceps
C. tissue forceps
C. tongue forceps
C.-Duval intestinal thumb forceps

Col•lins
C. umbilical clamp

col•loid
^{99m}Tc-sulfur c.
technetium-sulfur c.

col•lum *pl.* col•la
c. vesicae biliaris
c. vesicae felleae

Co•lo•CARE fe•cal oc•cult blood test

co•lo•ce•cos•to•my

co•lo•cen•te•sis

co•lo•cho•le•cys•tos•to•my

co•lo•cly•sis

co•lo•clys•ter

co•lo•co•lon•ic

co•lo•co•los•to•my

co•lo•cu•ta•ne•ous

co•lo•dys•pep•sia

co•lo•en•ter•ic

co•lo•en•ter•itis

co•lo•fix•a•tion

Col•o•gel

co•lo•hep•a•to•pexy

co•lo•il•e•al

co•lol•y•sis

co•lo•me•trom•e•ter

co•lon
c. ascendens
ascending c.
cathartic c.
c. descendens
descending c.
gangrenous c.
giant c.
iliac c.
irritable c.
lead-pipe c.
left c.
pelvic c.
pipestem c.
ptotic c.
right c.
sigmoid c.
c. sigmoideum
spastic c.
stovepipe c.
transverse c.
c. transversum

co•lon•al•gia

co•lon•ic

co•lo•ni•tis

col•o•ni•za•tion
bacterial c.

co•lono•fi•ber•scope

co•lo•nop•a•thy

co•lon•or•rha•gia

co•lono•scope
fiberoptic c.
Fujinon video c.
Machida FCS-ML II magnifying c.
Olympus CF-HM magnifying c.
Olympus CF-MB/LB c.
Olympus CF-MB-M magnifying c.
Olympus CF-UHM magnifying c.
Olympus SIF-M magnifying c.
Olympus video c.
ultrasound c.
Welch Allyn video c.

co•lono•scop•ic

co•lo•nos•co•pist

co•lo•nos•co•py
fiberoptic c.
index c.

co•lop•a•thy

co•lo•peri•ne•al

co•lo•pex•ia

co•lo•pex•ot•o•my

co•lo•pexy

Co•lo•plast pouch

co•lo•pli•ca•tion

co•lo•proc•tec•to•my

co•lo•proc•ti•tis

co•lo•proc•tos•to•my

co•lop•to•sis

co•lo•punc•ture

co•lo•rec•tal

co•lo•rec•ti•tis

co•lo•rec•tos•to•my

co•lo•rec•tum

co•lor•rha•phy

co•lor•rhea

co•lo•scope

co•los•co•py

Co•lo•Screen fe•cal oc•cult blood test

Co•lo•Screen tape

Co•lo•shield tube

co•lo•sig•moid•os•to•my

co•los•to•my
  ascending c.
  "blow-hole" c.
  decompressing c.
  descending c.
  distal c.
  diverting c.
  dry c.
  end c.
  end-descending c.
  end-loop c.
  Hartmann's c.
  ileotransverse c.
  loop c.
  loop transverse c.
  midline c.
  Mikulicz c.
  proximal c.
  sigmoid c.
  transrectus c.
  transverse c.
  wet c.

co•lot•o•my

co•lo•ure•ter•al

co•lo•uter•ine

co•lo•vag•i•nal

co•lo•ve•nous

co•lo•ves•i•cal

Colp
  C.-Hofmeister technique

col•po•rec•to•pexy

col•umn
  anal c's
  c's of Morgagni
  rectal c's

co•lum•na *pl.* co•lum•nae
  columnae anales
  columnae rectales [Morgagnii]

co•ly•pep•tic

co•ma
  hepatic c.

com•mu•ni•ca•tion
  horseshoe c.

com•part•ment
  inframesocolic c.

Com•pat En•ter•al De•liv•ery Sys•tem

Com•pat 199205 en•ter•al feed•ing pump

com•plaint
  summer c.

Com•pleat B tube feed•ing for•mu•la

Com•pleat Mod•i•fied tube feed•ing for•mu•la

Com•pleat Reg•u•lar Form tube feed•ing for•mu•la

com•ple•ment

com•plex
  AIDS-related c. (ARC)

com•plex *(continued)*
Carman-Kirklin meniscus c.
dorsal vagal c.
lactase-ceramidase c.
Meyenburg's c's
migrating myoelectric c.
rectal motor c.
urobilin c.
von Meyerberg c's

com•pli•ance
rectal c.

com•pres•sion
celiac axis c.
common bile duct c.
extramural common bile duct c.

ConA
concanavalin A

con•ca•nav•a•lin A

con•cre•tion
alvine c.

con•cus•sion
abdominal c., hydraulic

con•fig•u•ra•tion
cartwheel c.
J-pouch c.
rat-tail c.
W-pouch c.

con•ges•tion
hepatic c.

Con•go red

con•ju•gate
bilirubin c.
bilirubin ester c.
bilirubin protein c.

con•ju•ga•tion
c. of amino acids
c. of bilirubin

Con•nell
C. suture

Con•radi
C's line

con•scious•ness
colon c.

con•sis•ten•cy
food c.

Con•sti•lac

con•sti•pat•ed

con•sti•pa•tion
atonic c.
gastrojejunal c.
proctogenous c.
spastic c.

con•stric•tion
duodenopyloric c.

con•stric•tive

Con•stu•lose

con•tain•er
Safe-T-Flex enteral feeding c.
Travenol enteral feeding c.

con•ti•nence
fecal c.

con•trac•tion
Balli c.
Busi c.
Hirsch c.
Moultier c.
paradoxical puborectalis c. (PPC)
Payer-Strauss c.
Rossi c.
segmentation c.

con•trast
barium c.
bowel c.

Con•tro•lyte cal•o•rie sup•ple•ment

Cook
C's speculum

Coo•ley
DeBakey-C. retractor

Coons
C. guide
C./Carey endoprosthesis

Coop•er
C's hernia

Cope
C's clamp
C's sign

cop•per
c. thiocyanate

cop•ra•cra•sia

cop•rem•e•sis

cop•ro•lith

cop•ro•ma

cop•ro•por•phy•ria
erythropoietic c.
hereditary c.

cop•ro•por•phy•rin

cop•ro•sta•sis

cor•a•cid•i•um *pl.* cor•a•cid•ia

cord
hepatic c's

Cori
C. cycle

Co•ri•um

Crig•ler
C.-Najjar disease
C.-Najjar jaundice
C.-Najjar syndrome

co•ro•na•vi•rus

cor•pus *pl.* cor•po•ra
c. gastricum
c. pancreatis
c. ventriculare
c. ventriculi
c. vesicae biliaris

cor•pus *(continued)*
c. vesicae felleae

cor•pus•cle
Jaworski's c's

Cor•rec•tol

Cor•safe feed•ing tube

Cor•tef

Cor•ten•e•ma

Cor•ti•caine

cor•ti•co•ster•oid

cor•ti•co•tro•pin

Cor•ti•foam

cor•ti•sol

Cor•tro•phin-Zinc

Cos•me•gen

cos•tive

cos•tive•ness

Cot•a•zym

Cot•a•zym-65 B

Cot•a•zym-S

co•trans•port
sodium-bicarbonate c.
sodium-phosphate c.

Co•trim

co-tri•mox•a•zole

cot•ton
Oxycel c.

count
sponge c.
whole crypt mitotic c.

Cour•voi•si•er
C's gallbladder
C's law
C's sign
C.-Terrier syndrome

Cow•den
  C's disease
  C's syndrome

cox•sack•ie•vi•rus

CPH
  chronic persistent hepatitis

CR
  colon resection
  colorectal

Cra•foord
  C. thoracic scissors

cramp
  abdominal c.

cra•ter
  ulcer c.

CRC
  colorectal cancer
  colorectal carcinoma

Cream•a•lin

cre•a•tine

cre•at•i•nine

Cre•mer
  C. cannula

Cre•on

crep•i•tus

CREST syn•drome

Crile
  C. appendix clamp
  C. clamp
  C. gall duct forceps
  C. hemostat
  C. malleable retractor
  C. retractor
  C.-Wood needle holder

cri•sis *pl.* cri•ses
  hepatic c.

cri•te•ri•on *pl.* cri•te•ria
  Glasgow criteria (for severity of pancreatitis)
  Ranson criteria (for severity of pancreatitis)

Crit•i•care HN tube feed•ing for•mu•la

Crohn
  C's disease
  C's duodenitis

Crohn's Dis•ease Ac•tiv•i•ty In•dex

cro•mo•gly•cate

Cron•khite
  C.-Canada polyp
  C.-Canada syndrome

Cros•by
  C. capsule

CRS
  cherry red spot
  colon-rectal surgery
  colorectal surgery

crush•er
  Stetton spur c.
  Warthen spur c.

Cru•veil•hier
  C's disease
  C's ulcer
  C.-Baumgarten cirrhosis
  C.-Baumgarten syndrome

cryo•glob•u•lin•emia
  mixed c.

cryo•sur•gery

cryo•ther•a•py

crypt
  anal c's
  associated c.
  branched c.
  forked c.
  c's of Lieberkühn
  Luschka's c's

crypt *(continued)*
c. of Morgagni
mucous c's of duodenum

cryp•ta *pl.* cryp•tae
cryptae mucosae duodeni

cryp•ti•tis
anal c.

Cryp•to•coc•cus
C. neoformans

cryp•to•spo•rid•i•o•sis

Cryp•to•spo•ri•di•um

cryp•to•spo•ri•di•um

C&S
culture & sensitivity

CT
colon, transverse

C/TG
cholesterol/triglyceride (ratio)

CUC
chronic ulcerative colitis

Cub R-200 en•ter•al feed•ing pump

cuff
balloon c.

Cul•len
C's sign

cul•ture
stool c.

cup
ileostomy c.

curl•ing
esophageal c.

cur•rent
coagulating c.
cutting c.

Cursch•mann
C's disease

Cur•tis
Fitz-Hugh–C. syndrome

cur•va•tu•ra *pl.* cur•va•tu•rae
c. gastrica major
c. gastrica minor
c. ventriculi major
c. ventriculi minor

cur•va•ture
greater gastric c.
greater c. of stomach
lesser gastric c.
lesser c. of stomach

Cush•ing
C. forceps
C. suture
C's ulcer
C. vein retractor
C.-Rokitansky ulcer
Rokitansky-C. ulcer

cush•ion
anal c.

cy•a•no•co•bal•a•min

cy•a•no•sis
autotoxic c.
enterogenous c.

CYC
cyclophosphamide

Cyc
cyclophosphamide

cy•cla•cil•lin

cy•clase
adenylyl c.
guanyl c.
guanylyl c.

cy•cle
biliary c.
Cori c.
gastric c.
liver–adipose tissue c.
β-oxidation c.
Schiff's biliary c.

cy•cle *(continued)*
tricarboxylic acid c.
urea c.

cy•cli•zine

cy•clo•cyt•i•dine

cy•clo•oxy•gen•ase

cy•clo•phos•pha•mide

cy•clo•spor•ine

cy•pro•ter•one ac•e•tate

cyst
adventitious c.
alveolar hydatid c.
bile duct c.
choledochal c.
choledochus c.
chyle c.
compound c.
daughter c.
echinococcal c.
echinococcus c.
enteric c.
enterogenous c.
epidermoid c.
esophageal c.
false c.
gas c.
granddaughter c.
hepatic c.
hydatid c.
intraluminal c's
mesenteric c.
mother c.
multilocular c.
neoplastic c.
omental c's
pancreatic c.
sebaceous c.
secondary c.
solitary hepatic c.
sterile c.
unicameral c.
unilocular c.

cys•tad•e•no•car•ci•no•ma
biliary c.

cys•tad•e•no•car•ci•no•ma *(continued)*
hepatic c.

cys•tad•e•no•ma
biliary c.
hepatic c.

cys•ta•mine

cys•te•amine

cys•ti•cer•co•sis

Cys•ti•cer•cus
C. bovis
C. cellulosae

cys•ti•cer•cus *pl.* cys•ti•cer•ci

cys•ti•co•li•thec•to•my

cys•ti•co•li•tho•trip•sy

cys•ti•cor•rha•phy

cys•ti•cot•o•my

cys•tine

cys•tis *pl.* cys•ti•des
c. fellea

cys•to•du•o•de•nos•to•my

cys•to•en•tero•cele

cys•to•epip•lo•cele

cys•to•gas•tros•to•my

cys•to•je•ju•nos•to•my

Cys•to•spaz

Cys•to•spaz-M

cy•tar•a•bine

cy•to•chal•a•sin
c. B

cy•to•chrome
c. P-450

cy•to•chrome ox•i•dase

cy•to•chrome *c* ox•i•dase

cy•to•chrome b_5 re•duc•tase

cy•to•chrome P-450 re•duc•
tase

cy•to•ker•a•tin

cy•tol•o•gy
brush c.
exfoliative c.
salvage c.

cy•to•meg•a•lo•vi•rus

Cy•to•sar

Cy•to•tec

Cy•tox•an

Czer•ny
C. interrupted suture
C's suture
C.-Kocher-Perthes incision
C.-Lembert suture

D

D
daunorubicin

da•car•ba•zine

Da•co•dyl

Da•cron suture

DACT
dactinomycin

Dact
dactinomycin

dac•ti•no•my•cin

DAG
diacylglycerol

DALM
dysplasia-associated lesion or mass

dam
rubber d.

Dan•dy
D. nerve hook

dan•thron
d. and docusate

Dar•bid

Dar•i•con

DAT
diet as tolerated

dau•no•ru•bi•cin

Da•vid
D. rectal speculum
Vernon-D. proctoscope
Vernon-D. rectal speculum
Vernon-D. sigmoidoscope

Da•vid•off
D's cells

Da•vis
Rockey-D. incision

Da•vis *(continued)*
Rockey-D. modification of McBurney incision

Da•vol co•lon tube

Da•vol feed•ing bag

Da•vol feed•ing tube

Da•vy
Martin and D. speculum

DB
direct bilirubin

DBP
vitamin D–binding protein

DBW
desirable body weight

DC
descending colon
dilation catheter
duodenal cap

DCBE
double-contrast barium enema

DCC (deleted in colon carcinoma) gene

DD
digestive disease

DDP
cisplatin

Ddp
cisplatin

DE
duodenal exclusion

de Ala•mei•da
Hays-de A. gastric reservoir

Dean
- D.-MacDonald gastric resection clamp

death
- liver d.

Deav•er
- D's incision
- D. operating scissors
- D. retractor

De•Bak•ey
- DeB.-Cooley retractor

De•bray
- Housset-D. gastroscope

De•cho•lin

Dec•lo•my•cin

de•com•pres•sion
- biliary d.
- d. of bowel
- long intestinal tube d.

de•con•tam•i•na•tion
- intestinal d.
- selective bowel d.

DEF
- defecation

def
- defecation

def•e•ca•tion
- fragmentary d.

def•e•cog•ra•phy

de•fect
- acinar d.
- cobblestone filling d.
- filling d.
- mesenteric d.
- polypoid filling d.
- tailing d.

de•fi•cien•cy
- bile salt d.
- biotin d.
- calcium d.
- chromium d.

de•fi•cien•cy *(continued)*
- cobalamin d.
- copper d.
- disaccharidase d.
- essential fatty acid d.
- folate d.
- iron d.
- magnesium d.
- niacin d.
- nutritional d.
- potassium d.
- protein d.
- riboflavin d.
- sodium d.
- thiamine d.
- vitamin d.
- zinc d.

De•fi•col

de•form•a•bil•i•ty
- hepatic d.

de•form•i•ty
- crossbar d.

de•gen•er•a•tion
- ballooning d.
- feathery d.
- hepatolenticular d.

de•glu•ti•ble

de•glu•ti•tion

de•glu•ti•tive

de•glu•ti•to•ry

de•hy•dra•tion
- hyperosmotic nonketotic d.

de•hy•dro•bil•i•ru•bin

de•hy•dro•cho•lan•er•e•sis

de•hy•dro•cho•lic ac•id
- d.a. and docusate
- d.a., docusate, and phenolphthalein

de•hy•dro•em•e•tine

de•jec•ta

de•jec•tion

Del•ta-Cor•tef

De•Mar•tel
D. clamp
D.-Wolfson anastomosis clamp
D.-Wolfson clamp
D.-Wolfson clamp holder
D.-Wolfson closing forceps
Judd-D. gallbladder forceps
Zachary Cope-D. colon clamp

dem•e•clo•cy•cline

Dem•er•ol

4-de•meth•oxy•dau•no•ru•bi•cin (MGBG)

Den•nis
D. anastomosis clamp
D. clamp
D. intestinal forceps
D. and Varco operation

De-Nol

den•si•ty
nutrient d.

Den•ver shunt

de•oxy•cho•lan•er•e•sis

de•oxy•cho•late

de•oxy•chol•ic acid

de•oxy•doxo•ru•bi•cin

4-de•oxy•doxo•ru•bi•cin

de•oxy•guan•o•sine

de•oxy•ni•va•len•ol

de•pep•sin•ized

dep•Med•a•lone

De•po•ject

De•po-Med•rol

De•po•pred

De•po-Pred•ate

dep•o•si•tion
hyaline d.

de•riv•a•tive

Der•ma•lene su•ture

Der•ma•lon su•ture

DES
diffuse esophageal spasm

Des•champs
D. ligature needle

Des•jar•dins
D. gall duct probe
D. gallstone forceps
D. gallstone scoop

des•min

des•mo•some

de•sus•cep•tion

de•vas•cu•lar•iza•tion
hepatic d.

de•va•ze•pide

dex•a•meth•a•sone

Dex•on su•ture

dex•trin

dex•tro•gas•tria

dex•trose
d. and electrolytes

DG
diacylglycerol

DH
diaphragmatic hernia

DI
distal intestine

di•a•be•tes
d. mellitus (DM)

di•a•bro•sis

di•a•cho•re•ma

di•a•cho•re•sis

di•a•cyl•glyc•er•ol

di•ag•no•sis
- endoscopic d.

Di•a•lose

Di•a•lume

di•amine ox•i•dase

Di•a•mond
- D. tube

di•an•hy•dro•ga•lac•ti•tol

Di•ar-Aid

di•ar•rhea
- bile acid d.
- cachectic d.
- choleraic d.
- d. chylosa
- colliquative d.
- congenital chloride d.
- crapulous d.
- critical d.
- dientameba d.
- dysenteric d.
- enteral d.
- familial chloride d.
- fatty acid d.
- fermental d.
- fermentative d.
- flagellate d.
- gastrogenic d.
- hill d.
- inflammatory d.
- irritative d.
- lienteric d.
- mechanical d.
- morning d.
- mucous d.
- osmotic d.
- d. pancreatica
- pancreatogenous fatty d.
- paradoxical d.
- parenteral d.
- postvagotomy d.
- putrefactive d.

di•ar•rhea *(continued)*
- secretory d.
- serous d.
- stercoral d.
- toxigenic d.
- traveler's d.
- tropical d.
- tubercular d.
- virus d.
- watery d.
- white d.

di•ar•rhe•al

di•ar•rhe•ic

di•ar•rhe•o•gen•ic

Di•a•sorb

Di•a•tri•zo•ate-60

dia•tri•zo•ate
- d. meglumine
- d. sodium

di•az•e•pam

di•az•i•quone

Di•bent

di•both•rio•ceph•a•li•a•sis

Di•both•rio•ceph•a•lus

di•bro•mo•dul•ci•tol

2,5-di•bu•tyl-1,4-ben•zo•hy•dro•quin•one

Di•car•bo•sil

di•chlo•ro•metho•trex•ate

Dick•son
- D. osteotomy
- Ludwig-D.-MacDonald classification (for primary biliary cirrhosis)

di•clo•fe•nac

di•clox•a•cil•lin

di•cyc•lo•mine

Di-Cy•clo•nex

di•et
- cornstarch-rich d.
- defined-formula d.
- disease-specific d.
- elemental d.
- fructose-free d.
- galactose-free d.
- high fiber d.
- high-starch d.
- low available carbohydrate d.
- low fat d.
- low fiber d.
- low lactose d.
- low oxalate d.
- low-tyrosine/low-phenylalanine d.
- Sippy d.
- Travasorb hepatic d.
- Travasorb renal d.

di•e•tary

di•eth•yl•di•thio•car•ba•mate

Dieu•la•foy
- D's anomaly
- D's disease
- D's lesion
- D's triad
- D's ulcer
- D's vascular malformation

di•fen•ox•in
- d. and atropine

dif•fer•ence
- potential d.

Di-Gel

di•ges•tion

di•gly•co•al•de•hyde

di•hy•dro•pyr•i•dine

di•hy•droxy•alu•mi•num
- d. aminoacetate
- d. sodium carbonate

di•iso•pro•pyl imi•no•di•ace•tic ac•id

dil•a•ta•tion
- anal d.
- cecal d.
- gastric d.
- Lord's d.
- d. of the stomach
- toxic d. of bowel

di•la•tion
- balloon d.

di•la•tor
- American d.
- anal d.
- Backhaus d.
- Bakes d.
- balloon d.
- Barnes common duct d.
- bullet-tip d.
- Clark common duct d.
- Eder-Puestow d.
- Einhorn's d.
- Hurst d.
- Maloney d.
- mercury-filled d.
- olive-tipped d.
- Ottenheimer common duct d.
- Ramstedt pyloric stenosis d.
- Rapaport common duct d.
- Savary d.
- Savary-Gilliard d.
- Starck d.
- tapered-tip d.
- "through the scope" (TTS) d.
- Tucker d.

Di•lo•mine

di•meth•yl•hy•dra•zine

di•meth•yl•thio•urea

di•ni•trate

Di•oc•to

Di•oc•to-C

Di•oc•to-K

Dio•eze

di•os•mec•tite

Dio•suc•cin

Dio-Sul

Di•o•thron

Di•o•vol

Di•pen•tum

di•pep•tide

di•pep•ti•dyl ami•no•pep•ti•dase IV

Di•phe•na•tol

di•phen•i•dol

di•phen•oxy•late
 d. and atropine

di•phyl•lo•both•ri•a•sis

Di•phyl•lo•both•ri•i•dae

Di•phyl•lo•both•ri•um
 D. latum
 D. parvum
 D. taenioides

Di•py•lid•i•um
 D. caninum

di•py•rid•a•mole

di•rec•tion
 isoperistaltic d.

di•rec•tor
 grooved d.
 Larry rectal d.
 probe and groove d.

di•sac•cha•ri•dase

di•sac•cha•ride tri•pep•tide glyc•er•ol di•pal•mi•to•yl

Dis•an•throl

DISDA
 diisopropyl iminodiacetic acid

dis•ease (see also under *syndrome*)
 adult celiac d.
 adult polycystic d.
 Ajmalin liver d.
 alcohol-liver d.
 alcoholic liver d.
 Bassen-Kornzweig d.
 biliary tract d.
 Bouchard's d.
 Bradley's d.
 Brinton's d.
 Budd-Chiari d.
 Byler's d.
 Caroli's d.
 celiac d.
 Chagas' d.
 Chiari's d.
 cholesterol ester storage d.
 cholesteryl ester storage d. (CESD)
 chronic liver d.
 Cowden's d.
 Crigler-Najjar d.
 Crohn's d.
 Cruveilhier's d.
 Curschmann's d.
 cysticercus d.
 Dieulafoy's d.
 diffuse liver d.
 diverticular d.
 drug-induced liver d.
 Dubin-Sprinz d.
 echinococcus d.
 end-stage liver d.
 Fenwick's d.
 functional bowel d.
 gastroesophageal d.
 Gee-Thaysen d.
 Gilbert's d.
 glycogen storage d.
 graft-versus-host (GVH) d.
 Gross d.
 halothane-induced liver d.

dis•ease *(continued)*
- Hanot's d.
- hepatobiliary d.
- Heubner-Herter d.
- Hirschsprung's d.
- hydatid d., alveolar
- hydatid d., unilocular
- idiopathic inflammatory bowel d. (IIBD)
- immunoproliferative small intestine d.
- infantile celiac d.
- inflammatory bowel d.
- ischemic bowel d.
- Laënnec's d.
- Lane's d.
- Leyden's d.
- liver d.
- Ménétrier's d.
- metabolic liver d.
- noncommunicating polycystic d.
- pancreatic d.
- Patella's d.
- Payr's d.
- peptic d.
- peptic ulcer d. (PUD)
- polycystic liver d.
- rectal d.
- Rossbach's d.
- Ruysch's d.
- Schönlein-Henoch d.
- sigmoid diverticular d.
- Spencer's d.
- subacute liver d.
- Thaysen's d.
- tufting d.
- van den Bergh's d.
- veno-occlusive d. of the liver
- von Gierke's d.
- Whipple's d.
- Wilson's d.
- Wolman d.

Di•so•lan

Di•so•nate

dis•or•der
- defecation d.
- esophageal motility d.
- gastric motility d.

Di-So•sul

Di-Spaz

dis•place•ment
- fish-hook d.
- gallbladder d.

Disse
- D's spaces

dis•sec•tion
- flap d.
- lymph node d.
- pelvic d.
- sharp d.

dis•sec•tor
- Beaver d.
- MacDonald d.
- sponge d.

dis•ten•tion
- abdominal d.
- esophageal d.
- gastric d.
- intestinal d.
- intraluminal d.

di•ver•tic•u•li•tis
- perforating d.
- sigmoid d.

di•ver•tic•u•lo•sis
- bleeding d.
- esophageal intramural d.

di•ver•tic•u•lum *pl.* di•ver•tic•u•la
- colonic diverticula
- diverticula of colon
- epiphrenic d.
- esophageal d.
- false d.
- Ganser's d.
- giant d.
- Graser's d.
- d. ilei verum

di•ver•tic•u•lum *(continued)*
 intestinal d.
 Meckel's d.
 midesophageal d.
 pharyngeal d.
 pressure d.
 pulsion d.
 Rokitansky's d.
 supradiaphragmatic d.
 traction d.

Dix•on
 D.-Thomas-Smith colon clamp

DLC
 dual lumen catheter

DM
 duodenal mucosa

4-DMDR

DNR
 daunorubicin

Dnr
 daunorubicin

Dobb•hoff
 D. enteral feeding bag
 D. 8000 enteral feeding pump
 D. feeding tube

Do•cu•cal-P

Docu-K Plus

do•cu•sate
 bisacodyl and d.
 casanthranol and d.
 danthron and d.
 dehydrocholic acid and d.
 dehydrocholic acid, d., and phenolphthalein
 d. and phenolphthalein
 senna and d.

do•deca•dac•ty•li•tis

do•deca•dac•ty•lon

dol•i•cho•co•lon

dome
 Trask colostomy d.

dom•per•i•done

DON
 diazo-oxonorleucine

Don•na•gel-MB

Don•na•pec•to•lin-PG

Don•na•pine

Don•na-Sed

Don•na•tal

Don•na•tal No. 2

Don•phen

Don•na•gel-PG

Don•na•mor

do•pa

Dor•mia
 D. basket

Dot•ter
 Bilboa-D. tube

Dou•bi•let
 D. sphincterotome

dox•e•pin

Dox•i•dan

dox•i•flu•ri•dine

Dox•in•ate

doxo•ru•bi•cin

doxy•cy•cline

Doy•en
 D. abdominal scissors
 D's clamp
 D. cross action forceps
 D. intestinal clamp
 D. intestinal forceps
 D. raspatory and elevator
 D. straight intestinal forceps

DP
diminutive polyp

DR
diffuse redness

drain
Hemovac d.
Penrose d.
Pezzer d.
rubber d.

drain•age
biliary d.
button d.
continuous suction d.
endoscopic retrograde biliary d. (ERBD)
gravity d.
guided percutaneous d.
jejunal d. and biopsy
percutaneous d.
percutaneous transhepatic d.
percutaneous transhepatic biliary d.
T-tube d.
Wangensteen d.

Drei•ling
D. tube

drip
Murphy d.

Dro•sin
D's postures

Drum•mond
artery of D.
marginal artery of D.

DSMC Plus

D-S-S

DTIC
dacarbazine

Dtic
dacarbazine

DTIC-Dome

DTR
registered dietetic technician

DU
duodenal ulcer

Du•bin
D.-Johnson syndrome
D.-Sprinz disease
D.-Sprinz syndrome
Sprinz-D. syndrome

duct
Bernard's d.
bile d.
bile d., common
bile d's, interlobular
biliary d.
choledochous d.
common bile d.
cystic d.
extrahepatic bile d.
gall d.
d. of gallbladder
hepatic d., common
hepatic d., left
hepatic d., right
hepaticopancreatic d.
hepatocystic d.
Luschka's d's
pancreatic d.
pancreatic d., accessory
pancreatic d., minor
Rokitansky-Aschoff d's.
d. of Santorini
d. of Wirsung

duc•to•gram
pancreatic d.

duc•tog•ra•phy

duct•ule
bile d's
biliary d's
interlobular d's

duc•tu•lus *pl.* duc•tu•li
ductuli biliferi
ductuli interlobulares

duc•tus *pl.* duc•tus
d. biliaris
d. biliferi
d. choledochus
d. cysticus
d. hepaticus communis
d. hepaticus dexter
d. hepaticus sinister
d. interlobulares
d. lobi caudati dexter
d. lobi caudati sinister
d. pancreaticus
d. pancreaticus accessorius

Duf•field
D. deep surgery scissors

Du•ham•el
D. operation

Dukes
D. classification (for colorectal carcinoma)

Dul•co•dos

Dul•co•lax

Du•mon
D.-Gilliard prosthesis pushing tube

dump•ing

duod
duodenum

du•o•de•nal

du•o•de•nec•to•my

du•od•e•ni•tis
Crohn's d.
erosive d.

du•o•de•no•cho•lan•ge•itis

du•o•de•no•cho•le•cys•tos•to•my

du•o•de•no•cho•led•o•chot•o•my

du•o•de•no•col•ic

du•o•de•no•cys•tos•to•my

du•o•de•no•du•o•de•nos•to•my

du•o•de•no•en•ter•os•to•my

du•o•de•nog•ra•phy
hypotonic d.

du•o•de•no•he•pat•ic

du•o•de•no•il•e•os•to•my

du•o•de•no•je•ju•nos•to•my

du•o•de•nol•y•sis

du•o•de•no•pan•cre•a•tec•to•my

du•o•de•nor•rha•phy

du•o•de•no•scope
Fujinon video d.
Olympus video d.

du•o•de•no•scop•ic

du•o•de•nos•co•py

du•o•de•nos•to•my

du•o•de•not•o•my

du•o•de•num
inverted d.
mobile d.
redundant d.
supravaterian d.

Du•o•sol

Duo-Tube feed•ing tube

Du•pha•lac

du•pli•ca•tion
biliary tree d.

Du•puy•tren
D's suture

Du•ra•lone

Du•ra•morph

Du•val
Collin-D. intestinal thumb forceps
D. procedure

Du•val *(continued)*
D.-Allis tissue forceps

Du•ver•ney
D's foramen

Du•void

D&V
diarrhea and vomiting

Dy•cill

dye
hematoporphyrin derivative d. (HPD)
triazine d.

Dy•na•pen

dys•che•zia

dys•cho•lia

dys•en•ter•ic

dys•en•ter•i•form

dys•en•tery
amebic d.
bacillary d.
balantidial d.
bilharzial d.
catarrhal d.
ciliary d.
ciliate d.
epidemic d.
flagellate d.
Flexner's d.
fulminant d.
institutional d.
Japanese d.
malarial d.
malignant d.
protozoal d.
schistosomal d.
scorbutic d.
Sonne d.
spirillar d.
sporadic d.
viral d.

dys•func•tion
constitutional hepatic d.

dys•he•pa•tia

dys•ki•ne•sia
biliary d.

dys•pep•sia
acid d.
appendicular d.
appendix d.
catarrhal d.
cholelithic d.
colon d.
fermentative d.
flatulent d.
gastric d.
intestinal d.

dys•pep•tic

dys•per•i•stal•sis

dys•pha•gia
contractile ring d.
d. inflammatoria
d. lusoria
d. nervosa
d. paralytica
d. spastica
vallecular d.
d. valsalviana

dys•pha•gy

dys•pla•sia
arteriohepatic d.
colonic neuronal d.

dys•pra•gia
d. intermittens angiosclerotica intestinalis

dys•rhyth•mia
esophageal d.

dys•syn•er•gia
biliary d.

dys•tryp•sia

E

E
- enema
- enterococcus
- erosion
- esophagus

EA
- enteral alimentation
- enteroanastomosis

EAEC
- enteroadherent *Escherichia coli*

Earle
- E. rectal probe

EAS
- external anal sphincter

East•man
- E. cystic duct forceps

eat•ing
- binge e.

Ea•ton
- Chelsea-E. anal specula

EB
- esophageal body

E-Base

EBC
- esophageal balloon catheter

ebro•ti•dine

EC
- *Escherichia coli*
- esophageal carcinoma

echi•no•coc•ci•a•sis

echi•no•coc•co•sis

Echi•no•coc•cus
- *E. granulosus*

echi•no•coc•cus *pl.* echi•no•coc•ci

Echi•no•sto•ma

echo•en•do•scope

echo•vi•rus

Eck
- E's fistula

E. coli
- *Escherichia coli*

ec•ta•co•lia

ec•ta•sia
- vascular e.
- venous e.

ec•to•co•lon

ec•to•derm

ec•to•der•mal

ec•to•peri•to•ne•al

ec•to•peri•to•ni•tis

Eder
- E. gastroscope
- E.-Chamberlin gastroscope
- E.-Hufford gastroscope
- E.-Puestow dilator

Ed•lich
- E. tube

Ed•na
- E. towel clamp

Ed•ward•si•el•la
- *E. tarda*

EEA
- elemental enteral alimentation
- end-to-end anastomosis

EEA sta•pler

E.E.S.

EFA
essential fatty acids

EFC
endogenous fecal calcium

ef•face•ment
villous e.

Ef•fer-syl•li•um

EG
eosinophilic gastroenteritis
esophagogastrectomy

ega•grop•i•lus

EGD
esophagogastro-duodenos-copy

eges•ta

eges•tion

EGG
electrogastrogram
electrogastrography

EG (esophagogastric) junc•tion

EHBDA
extrahepatic bile duct atresia

EHC
enterohepatic circulation

EHEC
enterohemorrhagic *Escherichia coli*

EHO
extrahepatic obstruction

EHT (electrohydrothermal) co•ag•u•la•tion

EHT (electrohydrothermal) elec•trode

ei•co•sa•noid

EIEC
enteroinvasive *Escherichia coli*

Ein•horn
E's dilator
E. string test

Ei•sen•berg
E. catheter
E. torque guide

ejec•ta

elas•tase

Elas•ti•con

El•a•vil

elec•tro•cau•tery

elec•tro•co•ag•u•la•tion
bipolar e.
direct current e.
monopolar e.
multipolar e.

elec•trode
Buie fulguration e.
button e.
Cameron-Miller monopolar e.
concentric needle e.
EHT (electrohydrothermal) e.
Smith e.
suction e.

elec•tro•di•a•ther•my

elec•tro•ful•gur•a•tion

elec•tro•gas•tro•gram

elec•tro•gas•tro•graph

elec•tro•gas•trog•ra•phy

elec•tro•lyte
dextrose and e's

elec•tro•my•og•ra•phy
single-fiber e. (SFEMG)

elec•tro•phys•i•ol•o•gy
cellular e.
GI e.

elec•tro•sen•si•tiv•i•ty
mucosal e. (MES)

el•e•va•tor
Doyen raspatory and e.

El•li•ot
E's position

El•li•ott
E. gallbladder forceps

el•lip•tin•i•um ac•e•tate

El•lis
E.-van Creveld syndrome

El•li•son
Zollinger-E. syndrome
Zollinger-E. tumor

Ells•ner
E. gastroscope

El•spar

ELT
endoscopic laser therapy

EM
esophageal manometry

em•bo•li•za•tion
hepatic artery e.

EMD
esophageal mobility disorder

eme•sia

em•e•sis

em•e•ta•tro•phia

em•e•tine

Emex

EMG
electromyogram
electromyography

em•i•nence
caudate e. of liver

Emi•trip

em•phy•se•ma
intestinal e.

emp•ty•ing
delayed gastric e.
gastric e.
rapid gastric e.

em•py•e•ma
e. of gallbladder

emul•sion
lipid e.

Emul•soil

E-My•cin

EN
enema
enteral nutrition

enal•a•pril

En•care tube feed•ing for•mu•la

en•case•ment
pancreatic duct e.

en•ce•li•al•gia

en•ce•li•itis

en•ce•li•tis

en•ceph•a•lop•a•thy
bilirubin e.
hepatic e.

en•co•pre•sis

En•dep

en•do•ab•dom•i•nal

en•do•ap•pen•di•ci•tis

en•do•clip

en•do•co•li•tis

en•do•derm

en•do•der•mal

en•do•en•ter•itis

en•do•esoph•a•gi•tis

en•do•gas•tric

en•do•gas•tri•tis

en•do•grasp•er

en•do•her•ni•or•rha•phy

en•do•pep•ti•dase
- neutral e.
- pancreatic e's

en•do•peri•to•ne•al

en•do•peri•to•ni•tis

en•do•phle•bi•tis
- e. hepatica obliterans

en•do•pros•the•sis
- biliary e.
- Coons/Carey e.
- double pigtail e.
- Key-Med-Atkinson e.
- Medoc-Celestin e.
- peroral e.
- pigtail e.
- Procter-Livingstone e.
- straight e.
- Wilson-Cook e.

en•do•ra•dio•sonde

en•do•scis•sors

en•do•scope (see also specific types, e.g., *colonoscope*)
- ACMI e.
- CCD (charge-coupled device) e.
- double-channel e.
- fiberoptic e.
- flexible e.
- forward-viewing e.
- Fujinon UGI FP e.
- Fujinon video e.
- GIF XQ10 upper e.
- large-channel e.
- lateral-viewing e.
- Olympus GIF-2T e.

en•do•scope *(continued)*
- Olympus GIF-D2 e.
- Olympus GIF-P e.
- Olympus video e.
- rigid e.
- side-viewing e.
- therapeutic e.
- ultrasound e.
- Welch Allyn video e.

en•do•scop•ic

en•dos•co•pist

en•dos•co•py
- anal e.
- high-magnification e.
- infrared ray e.
- pediatric e.
- screening e.
- surveillance e.
- therapeutic e.
- transcolonic e.
- upper GI e.
- video e.

en•do•shears

en•do•so•no•graph•ic

en•do•so•nog•ra•phy

en•do•the•li•a•li•tis
- hepatic e.

en•do•tox•in

En•do-Tube feed•ing tube

en•e•ma *pl.* en•e•mas, e•nem•a•ta
- air contrast e.
- air-contrast barium e.
- barium e.
- blind e.
- cleansing e.
- contrast e.
- cromoglycate e.
- double contrast e.
- double-contrast barium e.
- Fleet e.
- high e.
- hydrocortisone e.

en·e·ma *(continued)*
- nutrient e.
- nutritive e.
- pancreatic e.
- phosphate e.
- saline e.
- sedative e.
- single-contrast barium e.
- small bowel e.
- soapsuds e.
- sodium polystyrene sulfonate e.
- starch e.
- tap water e.
- sodium phosphate and biphosphate e., sodium phosphate e.
- theophylline olamine e.

en·e·ma·tor

En·fa·mil for·mu·la

En·ger·ix-B

En·o·vil

en·pros·til

En·rich pro·tein and cal·o·rie sup·ple·ment

En·sure HN tube feed·ing for·mu·la

En·sure Plus HN tube feed·ing for·mu·la

En·sure Plus tube feed·ing for·mu·la

En·sure pro·tein and cal·o·rie sup·ple·ment

En·sure tube feed·ing for·mu·la

Ent·a·moe·ba
- *E. histolytica*

ENtech en·ter·al feed·ing pump

en·ter·ad·en

en·ter·ad·e·ni·tis

en·ter·al

en·ter·al·gia

en·ter·ec·ta·sis

en·ter·ec·to·my

en·ter·ic

en·ter·i·tis
- choleriform e.
- chronic cicatrizing e.
- e. cystica chronica
- diphtheritic e.
- *Escherichia coli* e.
- hemorrhagic e.
- e. gravis
- mucous e.
- e. necroticans
- e. nodularis
- phlegmonous e.
- e. polyposa
- protozoan e.
- pseudomembranous e.
- radiation e.
- regional e.
- segmental e.
- streptococcus e.
- terminal e.
- tuberculous e.

en·tero·anas·to·mo·sis

en·tero·bil·i·ary

En·tero·bi·us
- *E. vermicularis*

en·tero·cen·te·sis

en·tero·cho·le·cys·tost·o·my

en·tero·cho·le·cys·tot·o·my

en·tero·ci·ne·sia

en·tero·ci·net·ic

en·tero·clei·sis
- omental e.

en·ter·oc·ly·sis
- small bowel e.

En•ter•o•coc•cus
  E. fecalis

en•tero•co•lec•to•my

en•tero•co•li•tis
  antibiotic-associated e.
  hemorrhagic e.
  necrotizing e.
  pseudomembranous e.
  regional e.

en•tero•co•los•to•my

en•tero•cu•ta•ne•ous

en•tero•cyst

en•tero•cys•to•ma

en•tero•cyte

en•ter•odyn•ia

en•tero•en•ter•os•to•my

en•tero•gas•tric

en•tero•gas•tri•tis

en•ter•og•e•nous

en•tero•gram

en•tero•graph

en•ter•og•ra•phy

en•tero•he•pat•ic

en•tero•hep•a•ti•tis

en•tero•in•tes•ti•nal

en•tero•ki•nase

en•tero•ki•ne•sia

en•tero•ki•net•ic

en•tero•lith

en•tero•li•thi•a•sis

en•ter•ol•o•gy

en•ter•ol•y•sis

en•tero•me•ga•lia

en•tero•meg•a•ly

En•tero•mo•nas

en•tero•my•co•der•mi•tis

en•tero•my•co•sis
  e. bacteriacea

en•tero•my•ia•sis

en•ter•on

en•tero•ni•tis

en•tero•pa•re•sis

en•tero•path•o•gen

en•tero•patho•gen•e•sis

en•tero•path•o•gen•ic

en•ter•op•a•thy
  choleretic e.
  gluten e.
  HIV-1 (human
    immunodeficiency
    virus 1) e.
  protein-losing e.

en•tero•pexy

en•tero•plas•ty

en•tero•ple•gia

en•tero•pty•chia

en•tero•pty•chy

en•ter•or•rha•gia

en•ter•or•rha•phy
  circular e.

en•ter•or•rhea

en•ter•or•rhex•is

en•tero•scope

en•tero•sep•sis

en•tero•sorp•tion

en•tero•spasm

en•tero•sta•sis

en•tero•stax•is

en•tero•ste•no•sis

en•tero•sto•mal

en•ter•os•to•my
gun-barrel e.
tube e.

en•tero•tome

en•ter•ot•o•my

en•tero•tox•e•mia

en•tero•tox•in

en•tero•trop•ic

en•tero•ve•nous

en•tero•vi•rus

En•to•lase

En•tra•life HN tube feed•ing for•mu•la

En•tra•life tube feed•ing for•mu•la

En•tri•flex feed•ing tube

En•tri-HN feed•ing tube

En•tri-Pak en•ter•al feed•ing bag

En•tri-pak tube feed•ing for•mu•la

En•tri•tion-HN tube feed•ing for•mu•la

En•tri•tion tube feed•ing for•mu•la

EN•tube feed•ing tube

EN•tube-Pedi feed•ing tube

EN•tube Plus feed•ing tube

En•u•lose

en•zyme
angiotensin-converting e.
Cotazym pancreatic e's
Festal pancreatic e's
Ilozyme pancreatic es
Ku-Zyme HP pancreatic e's

en•zyme *(continued)*
Pancrease pancreatic e's
pancreatic e's
proteolytic e.
Viokase pancreatic e's

en•zy•mol•o•gy

eo•sin

EPEC
enteropathogenic *Escherichia coli*

epi•car•dia

epi•car•di•al

4′epi-doxo•ru•bi•cin

epi•gas•tral•gia

epi•gas•trog•ra•phy
impedance e.

epi•ge•net•ic

Epi•morph

epi•neph•rine

epip•lo•ec•to•my

epip•lo•ic

epip•lo•itis

epip•lo•on
great e.
lesser e.

epip•lo•pexy

epip•lo•plas•ty

epip•lor•rha•phy

epi•ru•bi•cin

epi•tha•lax•ia

ep•i•the•li•um *pl.* ep•i•the•lia
Barrett's e.
crypt e.
glandular e.
surface e.

epi•typh•li•tis

epi•typh•lon

E.P. My•cin

Ep•ping
  E. jaundice

Equa•lac•tin

Equi•let

ER
  epigastric region
  esophageal rupture

ERBD
  endoscopic retrograde biliary drainage

ERC
  endoscopic retrograde cholangiography

ERCP
  endoscopic retrograde cholangiopancreatogram
  endoscopic retrograde cholangiopancreatography

Er•ga•mi•sol

Er•lan•gen
  E. papillotome

ero•sion
  aphthous e.
  gastric e.
  mucosal e.

eruc•ta•tion

Er•yc

Ery•Ped

Ery-Tab

Eryth•ro

Eryth•ro•cin

Eryth•ro•cot

Eryth•ro•mid

eryth•ro•my•cin

Eryth•ro•zone

ES
  endoscopic sphincterotomy
  esophagus
  external sphincter

Esch
  Escherichia

Esch•e•rich•ia
  E. coli

ESI fi•ber•op•tic sig•moido•scope

ESO
  esophagoscopy
  esophagus

eso•gas•tri•tis

esoph•a•gal•gia

esoph•a•ge•al

esoph•a•gec•ta•sia

esoph•a•gec•ta•sis

esoph•a•gec•to•my

esoph•a•gism
  hiatal e.

esoph•a•gis•mus

esoph•a•gi•tis
  bacterial e.
  Candida e.
  chronic peptic e.
  corrosive e.
  e. dissecans superficialis
  drug-induced e.
  eosinophilic e.
  monilial e.
  pill e.
  radiation e.
  reflux e.
  stasis e.

esoph•a•go•car•dio•my•ot•o•my

esoph•a•go•cele

esoph•a•go•co•lo•gas•tros•to•my

esoph•a•go•co•lo•plas•ty

esoph•a•go•du•o•de•nos•to•my

esoph•a•go•dyn•ia

esoph•a•go•en•ter•os•to•my

esoph•a•go•esoph•a•gos•to•my

esoph•a•go•fun•do•pexy

esoph•a•go•gas•trec•to•my

esoph•a•go•gas•tric

esoph•a•go•gas•tro•anas•to•mo•sis

esoph•a•go•gas•tro•du•o•de•nos•co•py

esoph•a•go•gas•tro•my•ot•o•my

esoph•a•go•gas•tro•pexy
  intercostal pedicle e.

esoph•a•go•gas•tro•plas•ty

esoph•a•go•gas•tros•co•py

esoph•a•go•gas•tros•to•my
  Abbott e.
  Barrett e.
  Clagett-Barrett e.
  Johnson e.
  Thal e.
  Woodward e.

esoph•a•go•gram
  double channel e.
  solid-column e.
  tube e.

esoph•a•go•je•ju•no•gas•tros•to•mo•sis

esoph•a•go•je•ju•no•gas•tros•to•my

esoph•a•go•je•ju•no•plas•ty

esoph•a•go•je•ju•nos•to•my

esoph•a•gol•o•gy

esoph•a•go•ma•la•cia

esoph•a•go•my•co•sis

esoph•a•go•my•ot•o•my
  Heller's e.

esoph•a•go•plas•ty

esoph•a•go•pli•ca•tion

esoph•a•gop•to•sis

esoph•a•go•res•pi•ra•to•ry

esoph•a•go•scope

esoph•a•gos•co•py

esoph•a•go•spasm

esoph•a•go•ste•no•sis

esoph•a•gos•to•ma

esoph•a•gos•to•my

esoph•a•go•tome

esoph•a•got•o•my

esoph•a•gus
  Barrett's e.
  nutcracker e.

eso•ru•bi•cin

Es•po•tabs

es•ter
  cholesteryl e.
  phthalate e's

ESV
  esophageal valve

ESWL
  extracorporeal shock wave lithotripsy

ET
  endotracheal tube
  enterostomal therapy

état
  é. mammelonné

ETEC
  enterotoxic *Escherichia coli*
  enterotoxigenic *Escherichia coli*

eth•a•nol
  e. oleate

Eth•i•bond su•ture

Eth•i•lon su•ture

ethi•o•fos

Ethox feed•ing tube

Ethox/Bar•ron 2000 Feed•ing Pump Sys•tem

Eth•ril

Eth•y•ol

ETOP
  etoposide

eto•po•side (VP-16)

eu•chlor•hy•dria

eu•cho•lia

eu•chyl•ia

eu•pan•cre•a•tism

eu•pep•sia

eu•pep•sy

eu•pep•tic

eu•peri•stal•sis

EUS
  endoscopic ultrasonography

evac•u•a•tion
  rectal e.

Evac-U-Gen

Evac-U-Lax

Ev•ans
  E. blue

even•tra•tion

Ev•er•ett
  E. pile forceps

evis•cer•a•tion

E-Vis•ta

EVS
  esophageal variceal sclerotherapy

Ewald
  E's node
  E. tube

ex•am•i•na•tion
  anorectal e.
  bidigital e.
  digital e.
  parasite e.
  peroral pneumocolon e.
  reflux small bowel e.
  retrograde small bowel e.

ex•change
  chloride-bicarbonate e.
  sister chromatid e.
  sodium-calcium e.
  sodium-hydrogen e.

ex•ci•sion
  cloverleaf e. of hemorrhoids
  full-thickness local e.
  transanal e.

ex•cre•ment

ex•cre•men•ti•tious

ex•cres•cence
  polypoid e.

ex•cre•tion
  biliary e.

ex•en•din

ex•en•ter•itis

Ex-Lax

exo•co•li•tis

exo•en•zyme
e.-S

exo•gas•tric

exo•gas•tri•tis

exo•pep•ti•dase
pancreatic e's

exo•phyt•ic

ex•pen•di•ture
resting energy e. (REE)

ex•tra•co•lon•ic

ex•tract
malt soup e. and psyllium

ex•trac•tion
stone e.

ex•tra•he•pat•ic

ex•tra•pan•cre•at•ic

ex•tra•peri•to•ne•al

ex•trav•a•sate
bile e.

ex•u•date
fibrinous e.

eye•let

EZ CAT

F

F
  fat
  fecal

FA
  fatty acid

face•plate

fa•ci•es *pl.* fa•ci•es
  f. abdominalis
  f. anterior pancreatis
  f. diaphragmatica hepatis
  f. hepatica
  f. inferior hepatis
  f. inferior pancreatis
  f. posterior hepatis
  f. posterior pancreatis
  f. superior hepatis
  f. visceralis hepatis

fac•tor
  acid-inhibitory f.
  gastric inhibitor f.
  hepatocyte growth f.
  insulin-like growth f's (IGF)
  f. VIII

fail•ure
  acute hepatic f.
  fulminant hepatic f.
  liver f.

Falk
  F. appendectomy spoon

FAM
  fluorouracil, doxorubicin, and mitomycin C

FAMe
  5-fluorouracil, doxorubicin, and semustine

FAMMM (familial atypical multiple mole melanoma) syn•drome

fa•mo•ti•dine

Fans•ler
  F. anoscope

FAP
  familial adenomatous polyposis

fas•cia *pl.* fas•ciae
  abdominal f., internal
  anal f.
  f. of Camper
  Camper's f.
  fasciae of colon
  f. diaphragmatis pelvis inferior
  f. diaphragmatis pelvis superior
  endoabdominal f.
  esophagophrenic f.
  extraperitoneal f.
  f. extraperitonealis
  fusion f.
  ischiorectal f.
  pelvic f., visceral
  f. pelvis visceralis
  rectal f.
  rectovesical f.
  rectus f.
  subperitoneal f.
  f. subperitonealis
  f. transversalis
  visceral f. of pelvis
  Waldeyer's f.

fas•cic•u•lus *pl.* fas•cic•u•li
  longitudinal fasciculi of colon

Fas•ci•o•la
  F. gigantica
  F. hepatica

fas•cio•li•a•sis

Fas•ci•o•loi•des
  F. magna

fas•ci•o•lop•si•a•sis

Fas•ci•o•lop•sis
F. buski

fast•ing
intermediate f.
partial f.
prolonged f.
total f.

fat
dietary f.
fecal f.
ischiorectal f.
perirectal f.
properitoneal f.
submucosal f.

fat•ty ac•id
essential f.a.
esterified f.a.
free f.a's (FFA)
hydroxy f.a.
medium-chain f.a. (MCFA)
monounsaturated f.a's
nonesterified f.a's (NEFA)
polyunsaturated f.a's
saturated f.a's
short-chain f.a. (SCFA)
unsaturated f.a's

FCC
familial colon cancer

fe•cal

fe•ca•lith

fe•ca•lo•ma

fe•ces

fec•u•lent

Fe•de•ri•ci
F's sign

fe•do•to•zine

feed•ing
enteral f.
infant f.
nasogastric tube f.

feed•ing *(continued)*
sham f.
transitional f.
tube f.

Feen-a-Mint

Feh•land
F. right angle colon clamp

Fen•ger
F. gallstone probe
F. spiral gallstone forceps

Fen•wick
F's disease

Fer•gu•son
F. abdominal scissors
F. anal retractor
F. anoscope
F. gallstone scoop
F. needle
F. technique
F. tenaculum forceps
F.-Moon rectal retractor
Hill-F. rectal retractor
Hill-F. retractor

fer•men•ta•tion

Fer•ris
F. common duct scoop

fer•ri•tin
serum f.

Fes•tal II

Fes•tal pan•cre•at•ic en•zymes

fe•tor
f. hepaticus

fe•ver
Charcot's f.
intermittent hepatic f.

FF
fat free
fecal frequency

FFE
fecal fat excretion

FFS
fat-free supper

fi•ber
dietary f.
oblique gastric f's
oblique f's of stomach

Fi•ber•all

fi•ber•co•lono•scope

Fi•ber•Con

fi•ber•gas•tro•scope

fi•ber•scope
gastrointestinal f.
Hirschowitz gastroduodenal f.
Olympus GF-EU1 gastrointestinal f.
pediatric f.

fi•bra *pl.* fi•brae
fibrae obliquae gastricae
fibrae obliquae ventriculi

fi•bro•ma•to•sis
f. ventriculi

fi•bro•sar•co•ma

fi•bro•sis
acholangic biliary f.
anal f.
biliary f.
congenital hepatic f.
cystic f.
hepatic f.
periportal f.

field
anterior-posterior f.
lateral f.
posterior-anterior f.

film
plain f.
spot f.

Fine
Myers and F. test

Fin•ney
F's operation
F. pyloroplasty
F. strictureplasty
Grondahl-F. operation
von Haberer-F. technique

Fin•ster•er
Hofmeister-F. technique

First•Choice Drain•able Pouch

Fisch•er
Neubauer and F's test

fis•su•ra *pl.* fis•su•rae
f. in ano
f. ligamenti teretis
f. ligamenti venosi

fis•sure
anal f.
anterior f.
f. in ano
f. for ligamentum teres
f. for ligamentum venosum
longitudinal f.
portal f.
posterior f.
f. of round ligament
sagittal f. of liver
transverse f.
umbilical f.

fis•sur•ec•to•my

fis•tu•la *pl.* fis•tu•lae, fis•tu•las
abdominal f.
anal f.
f. in ano
anterior f.
biliary f.
biliary-enteric f.
f. bimucosa
blind f.
f. cibalis
colocolonic f.
coloenteric f.
colonic f.
coloperineal f.

fis•tu•la *(continued)*
colouretral f.
colouterine f.
colovaginal f.
colovenous f.
colovesical f.
Eck's f.
esophagopulmonary f.
esophagorespiratory f.
external f.
extrasphincteric f.
fecal f.
gastric f.
hepatic f.
horseshoe f.
H-type f.
internal f.
intestinal f.
intrasphincteric f.
mucous f.
pancreatic f.
perianal f.
stercoral f.
Thiry-Vella f.
transphincteric f.
umbilical f.
Vella's f.

fis•tu•li•za•tion

fis•tu•lo•en•ter•os•to•my

Fitz-Hugh
F.–Curtis syndrome

fix•a•tion
tissue f.

FJP
familial juvenile polyposis

FL
fatty liver
full liquid (diet)

Flag•yl

flat•u•lence

flat•u•lent

Fla•tu•lex

fla•tus

fla•vone

FLC
fatty liver cell

Fleet Ba•by•lax

Fleet Bis•ac•o•dyl

Fleet Bis•ac•o•dyl Prep

Fleet En•e•ma

Fleet En•e•ma Min•er•al Oil

Fleet Fla•vored Cas•tor Oil

Fleet Phos•pho-So•da

Flet•cher's Cas•tor•ia

fleur•ette

Flex•i•cal Cit•ro•tein pro•tein and cal•o•rie sup•ple•ment

Flex•i•flo Com•pan•ion en•ter•al feed•ing pump

Flex•i•flo en•ter•al feed•ing pump

Flex•i•flo II en•ter•al feed•ing pump

Flex•i•flo III en•ter•al feed•ing pump

Flex•i•flo Top-Fill En•ter•al Nu•tri•tion Sys•tem

Flexi-Flow feed•ing tube

Flex•ner
F's dysentery

flex•u•ra *pl.* flex•u•rae
f. coli dextra
f. coli sinistra
f. duodeni inferior
f. duodeni superior
f. duodenojejunalis
f. hepatica coli
f. lienalis coli
f. perinealis recti

flex•u•ra *(continued)*
f. sacralis recti

flex•ure
duodenojejunal f.
hepatic f. of colon
inferior f. of duodenum
left colic f.
left f. of colon
perineal f. of rectum
right colic f.
right f. of colon
sacral f. of rectum
sigmoid f.
splenic f. of colon
superior f. of duodenum

FLKS
fatty liver and kidney syndrome

floc•cu•late
calcific f.

floc•cu•lus *pl.* floc•cu•li
calcific f.

Flo•gard 2000 en•ter•al feed•ing pump

floor
pelvic f.

flo•ra
intestinal f.

flow
bile f.
gastric mucosal blood f.
hepatic blood f.
intestinal blood f.
mucosal blood f.
pancreatic blood f.
splanchnic blood f.

flow•me•ter

Flow-Thru feed•ing tube

flox•uri•dine

flu•co•na•zole

flu•dar•a•bine
f. phosphate

flu•id
ascitic f.

fluke
intestinal f's
liver f's

flu•ma•zen•il

flu•me•cin•ol

flu•o•ro•do•pan

flu•o•ro•meth•o•lone

flu•o•ro•scope
C-arm f.

flu•o•ros•co•py

flu•o•ro•ura•cil

5-flu•o•ro•ura•cil

flur•bip•ro•fen

flush
colonic f.

flux
celiac f.

FNA
fine-needle aspiration

FNAB
fine-needle aspiration biopsy

FNB
fine needle biopsy

FNTHC
fine-needle transhepatic cholangiography

FOBT
fecal occult blood test

Fo•gar•ty
F. balloon
F. biliary probe
F. catheter
F. Hydrogrip clamp

fo•late
  red blood cell f.
  serum f.

fold
  cecal f's
  cholecystoduodenocolic f.
  circular f's
  circular f's of Kerckring
  costocolic f.
  duodenojejunal f.
  duodenomesocolic f.
  gastric f's
  gastropancreatic f., left
  gastropancreatic f., right
  Heister's f.
  Hensing's f.
  hepatopancreatic f.
  horizontal f's of rectum
  ileocecal f.
  ileocolic f.
  inferior duodenal f.
  Kerckring's f's (of small intestine)
  Kohlrausch's f's
  f's of large intestine
  longitudinal f. of duodenum
  mucous f's of rectum
  Nélaton's f.
  pancreaticogastric f., left
  paraduodenal f.
  parietocolic f.
  rectal f's
  semilunar f's of colon
  semilunar f. of transversalis fascia
  sentinel f.
  sigmoid f's of colon
  spiral f.
  spiral f. of cystic duct
  superior duodenal f.
  transverse f's of rectum
  Treves' f.
  vascular cecal f.
  villous f's of stomach

Fo•ley
  F. bag catheter

fol•li•cle
  gastric f's
  intestinal f's
  Lieberkühn's f's
  lymph f.
  solitary f's

fol•lic•u•lus *pl.* fol•lic•u•li
  f. lymphaticus
  folliculi lymphatici aggregati
  folliculi lymphatici gastrici
  folliculi lymphatici recti
  folliculi lymphatici solitarii
  folliculi lymphatici splenici

fo•ra•men *pl.* fo•ra•mi•na
  Duverney's f.
  epiploic f.
  f. epiploicum
  omental f.
  f. omentale
  f. of Winslow

for•ceps
  Adair tissue-holding f.
  Adson f.
  Adson-Brown f.
  alligator f.
  Allis f.
  Allis tissue f.
  Allis-Adair tissue f.
  Babcock f.
  Babcock intestinal f.
  Bainbridge intestinal f.
  Barrett intestinal f.
  Barrett-Murphy intestinal thumb f.
  basket f.
  bayonet f.
  Beardsley intestinal f.
  Beck aorta f.
  Beebe hemostatic f.
  Bevan gallbladder f.
  biopsy f.

for•ceps *(continued)*
- Blalock pulmonary artery f.
- Blanchard hemorrhoid f.
- Bonney dissecting f.
- Bozeman f.
- Bridge deep surgery f.
- Brunner intestinal f.
- Brunner tissue f.
- Buie biopsy f.
- Child intestinal f.
- Children's Hospital intestinal f.
- clip applying f.
- Collin intestinal f.
- Collin tissue f.
- Collin tongue f.
- Collin-Duval intestinal thumb f.
- Crile gall duct f.
- curved mosquito f.
- Cushing f.
- DeMartel-Wolfson closing f.
- Dennis intestinal f.
- Desjardins gallstone f.
- double-spoon biopsy f.
- Doyen cross action f.
- Doyen intestinal f.
- Doyen straight intestinal f.
- Duval-Allis tissue f.
- Eastman cystic duct f.
- Elliott gallbladder f.
- Everett pile f.
- Fenger spiral gallstone f.
- Ferguson tenaculum f.
- foreign body f.
- Foss clamp f.
- Foss intestinal clamp f.
- Frankfeldt grasping f.
- gallstone f.
- Gavin-Miller intestinal f.
- Gavin-Miller tissue f.
- Gilbert cystic duct f.
- Gold deep surgery f.
- Gray cystic duct f.

for•ceps *(continued)*
- Gray gallbladder traction f.
- Green cystic duct f.
- Hamilton deep surgery f.
- Harrington f.
- Healy GI f.
- Hirschman hemorrhoidal f.
- hot-biopsy f.
- Hoyt deep surgery f.
- Jackson biopsy f.
- Johns Hopkins gallbladder f.
- Judd-Allis intestinal f.
- Judd-DeMartel gallbladder f.
- Kelly-Murphy f.
- Kelly-Murphy f., curved
- Kent deep surgery f.
- Kocher f.
- Kocher intestinal f.
- Lahey gall duct f.
- Lahey-Babcock f.
- Lane f.
- Lane dissecting f.
- Lane tissue f.
- Lawrence deep surgery f.
- Leonard deep surgery f.
- Lockwood intestinal f.
- Lockwood-Allis tissue f.
- Lovelace f.
- Lower gall duct f.
- McKenzie clip-applying f.
- Martin f.
- Mayo-Robson gastrointestinal f.
- Meeker deep surgery f.
- Metzenbaum f.
- Michigan intestinal f.
- Mixter f.
- mosquito f.
- Moynihan artery f.
- Moynihan gallbladder f.
- Moynihan gall duct f.
- Moynihan skin f.
- Ochsner f.
- Olympus hot biopsy f.

for•ceps *(continued)*
- Parker-Kerr f.
- Péan's f.
- Péan artery f.
- Péan GI f.
- Péan grasping f.
- peanut sponge f.
- Pemberton anastomosis f.
- Pennington hemorrhoidal f.
- Percy intestinal f.
- Percy tissue f.
- plain f.
- Porter duodenal f.
- Potts anastomosis f.
- Potts-Smith f.
- Potts-Smith mouse-tooth tissue f.
- Potts-Smith tissue f.
- Rampley sponge holding f.
- Randall stone f.
- Ratliff-Blake gallstone f.
- Ratliff-Mayo gallstone f.
- rectal alligator biopsy f.
- Richmond thumb tissue f.
- Robbers f.
- Rochester gallstone f.
- Rochester-Ochsner f.
- Rochester-Péan f.
- Rugby deep surgery f.
- Russian f.
- Schnidt gall duct f.
- Schoenberg intestinal f.
- Scudder intestinal f.
- Shallcross cystic duct f.
- sigmoidoscopic biopsy f.
- Smith f.
- Snyder deep surgery f.
- Spencer Wells f.
- spike f.
- sponge f.
- sponge-holding f.
- stone f.
- Stone closing f.
- stone-crushing f.
- stone-holding f.
- Storey gall duct f.
- straight mosquito f.

for•ceps *(continued)*
- Thoms-Allis tissue f.
- Thorek-Mixter gallbladder f.
- three-pronged grasping f.
- thumb f.
- tissue f.
- tissue mouse-tooth f.
- tongue f.
- toothed f.
- Turrell angulated specimen f.
- Varco gallbladder f.
- Wells thumb tissue f.
- Williams intestinal f.
- Williams tissue f.
- Yeomans rectal biopsy f.

For•ma•cath cath•e•ter

for•ma•tion
- bile acid–dependent bile f.
- bile acid–independent bile f.
- gallstone f.
- Gothic arch f.

for•mu•la *pl.* for•mu•lae, for•mu•las
- Amin-Aid renal f.
- Attain tube feeding f.
- Besure tube feeding f.
- blenderized food f.
- Citrotein tube feeding f.
- Compleat B tube feeding f.
- Compleat Modified tube feeding f.
- Compleat Regular Form tube feeding f.
- Criticare HN tube feeding f.
- Encare tube feeding f.
- Enfamil f.
- Ensure HN tube feeding f.
- Ensure Plus HN tube feeding f.
- Ensure Plus tube feeding f.
- Ensure tube feeding f.

for•mu•la *(continued)*
Entralife HN tube feeding f.
Entralife tube feeding f.
Entrapack tube feeding f.
Entri-pak tube feeding f.
Entrition-HN tube feeding f.
Entrition tube feeding f.
Formula 2 tube feeding f.
hepatic f.
Hepatic-Aid hepatic f.
Isocal HCN tube feeding f.
Isocal tube feeding f.
Isofiber tube feeding f.
Isomil f.
Isotein HN tube feeding f.
Jevity tube feeding f.
Lofenalac f.
Meritene tube feeding f.
MSUD f.
Newtrition tube feeding f.
Nursoy f.
Nutramigen f.
Nutren 1.0 tube feeding f.
Nutren 1.5 tube feeding f.
Nutren 2.0 tube feeding f.
Osmolite HN tube feeding f.
Osmolite tube feeding f.
Peptamen tube feeding f.
Pepti-2000 tube feeding f.
Portagen f.
Pre-Attain tube feeding f.
Precision Isotonic tube feeding f.
Precision LR tube feeding f.
Pregestimil f.
Premature Enfamil f.
ProFiber tube feeding f.
ProSobee f.
Protamin tube feeding f.
Pulmocare tube feeding f.
RCF f.
Reabilan HN tube feeding f.
Reabilan tube feeding f.

for•mu•la *(continued)*
renal f.
Replete tube feeding f.
Resource tube feeding f.
S-14 f.
Similac f.
Similac Special Care f.
SMA f.
stress f.
Stresstein TEN stress f.
Sustacal tube feeding f.
TEN tube feeding f.
Tolerex tube feeding f.
Traum-Aid HBC stress f.
TraumaCal tube feeding f.
Travasorb HN tube feeding f.
Travasorb MCT tube feeding f.
Travasorb STD tube feeding f.
Travasorb tube feeding f.
Vital tube feeding f.
Vitaneed tube feeding f.
Vivonex TEN stress f.

For•mu•la 2 tube feed•ing for•mu•la

For•mu•lex

for•nix *pl.* for•ni•ces
gastric f.
f. gastricus
f. of stomach
f. ventricularis
f. ventriculi

Foss
F. anterior resection clamp
F. clamp forceps
F. gallbladder retractor
F. intestinal clamp forceps

fos•sa *pl.* fos•sae
Broesike's f.
f. caecalis
crural f.
f. cystidis felleae
digital f., inferior

fos•sa *(continued)*
- duodenal f., inferior
- duodenal f., superior
- duodenojejunal f.
- femoral f.
- f. of gallbladder
- Gruber-Landzert f.
- ileocecal f., inferior
- ileocecal f., superior
- ileocolic f.
- infraduodenal f.
- f. intermesocolica transversa
- intersigmoid f.
- ischiorectal f.
- f. of Jonnesco
- Landzert's f.
- f. for ligamentum teres
- longitudinal fossae of liver, right
- f. longitudinalis hepatis
- Luschka's f.
- mesentericoparietal f.
- mesogastric f.
- f. of omental sac, inferior
- f. of omental sac, superior
- paraduodenal f.
- parajejunal f.
- retrocecal f.
- retroduodenal f.
- fossae sagittales dextrae hepatis
- fossae sagittales hepatis
- f. sagittalis sinistra hepatis
- splenic f. of omental sac
- subcecal f.
- subsigmoid f.
- f. transversalis hepatis
- f. of Treitz
- f. umbilicalis hepatis
- f. venae cavae
- f. venae umbilicalis
- f. vesicae felleae
- Waldeyer's f.

Fou•chet
- F's reagent

Fou•chet *(continued)*
- F's test

fo•vea *pl.* fo•veae
- crural f.
- femoral f.

fo•ve•o•la *pl.* fo•ve•o•lae
- foveolae gastricae

Fow•ler
- F.-Weir incision

FP
- food poisoning

FPC
- familial polyposis coli

Fr
- French scale

Frank
- F's operation
- Ssabanejew-F. operation

Frank•feldt
- F. grasping forceps
- F. hemorrhoidal needle
- F. rectal snare

Frank•lin
- F. flexible retractor
- F.-Silverman biopsy cannula

Fred•er•ick Mill•er feed•ing tube

Fre•det
- F.-Ramstedt operation
- F.-Ramstedt pyloromyotomy

Frei•burg bi•op•sy set

French
- F. eye needle
- F. scale

fren•u•lum *pl.* fren•u•la
- f. of ileocecal valve
- f. valvae ilealis
- f. valvae ileocaecalis

fre•num *pl.* fre•na
f. of Morgagni

fre•quen•cy
bowel f.
stool f.

Fritsch
F's retractor

Frosst•image HIDA

Frosst•image MAA

Frosst•image Sul•fur Col•loid

Frost•berg
F's reversed 3 sign

fruc•tose

fruc•tose al•do•lase

fruc•tose al•do•lase de•fi•cien•cy

fruc•tose di•phos•pha•tase

fruc•tose di•phos•pha•tase de•fi•cien•cy

Fryk•man
F.-Goldberg procedure

FTLE
full-thickness local excision

Ftor•a•fur

5-FU
5-fluorouracil

FUDR
5-fluorouracil deoxyribonucleoside

Fu•ji•non PRO-PC fi•ber•op•tic sig•moido•scope

Fu•ji•non SIG-E2 fi•ber•op•tic sig•moido•scope

Fu•ji•non SIG-PC fi•ber•op•tic sig•moido•scope

Fu•ji•non UGI FP en•do•scope

Fu•ji•non vi•deo co•lono•scope

Fu•ji•non vi•deo du•o•de•no•scope

Fu•ji•non vi•deo en•do•scope

Ful•ton
F. deep surgery scissors

func•tion
secretory f.

fun•do•pli•ca•tion
Belsey 270° f.
Nissen f.
Toupet f.

fun•dus *pl.* fun•di
f. of gallbladder
gastric f.
f. gastricus
f. of stomach
f. ventricularis
f. ventriculi
f. vesicae biliaris
f. vesicae felleae

fu•nic•u•lus *pl.* fu•nic•u•li
hepatic f.

fu•ra•zol•i•done

Fur•niss
F. anastomosis clamp
F.-Clute clamp
F.-Clute duodenal clamp

fu•ro•sem•ide

Fur•ox•one

fur•row
Liebermeister's f's

G

G
  gastrin
  glycogen

G+
  gram positive

G−
  gram negative

GA
  gastric antrum

Ga•bri•el
  G. proctoscope

Ga•ca•vit

gad•o•lin•i•um-eth•oxy•benz•yl-DTPA

GAG
  glycosaminoglycan

ga•lac•ti•tol

ga•lac•to•pex•ic

ga•lac•to•pexy

ga•lac•tose

ga•lac•tos•emia
  Indiana variant g.
  Los Angeles variant g.
  Rennes variant g.

ga•lac•to•si•dase

β-D-ga•lac•to•side ga•lac•to•hy•dro•lase

ga•lac•to•syl•trans•fer•ase

ga•lan•in

Gal•e•a•ti
  G's glands

gall

gall•blad•der
  bifid g.
  bilobed g.

gall•blad•der *(continued)*
  Courvoisier's g.
  fish-scale g.
  floating g.
  hourglass g.
  mobile g.
  multiseptate g.
  sandpaper g.
  stasis g.
  strawberry g.
  wandering g.

Gal•lie
  G. transplant

gall•stone
  black g.
  brown g.
  cholesterol g.
  pigment g.
  unextractable g.

GALT
  gut-associated lymphatic tissue
  gut-associated lymphoid tissue

Gam•bee
  G. anastomosis
  G. stitch

gam•ma glu•ta•myl trans•fer•ase (GGT)

gam•ma glu•ta•myl trans•pep•ti•dase

gam•ma-hy•droxy•bu•ty•rate

gan•ci•clo•vir

Gan•ser
  G's diverticulum

Gant
  G's clamp

Gan•tan•ol

Ga•ra•my•cin

Gard•ner
G's syndrome

Gar•lock
G's incision

GAS
gastroenterology

gas
intestinal g.

Gas-is-gon

Gas Re•lief

gas•ter

gas•tral•go•ke•no•sis

gas•tra•tro•phia

gas•trec•to•my
partial g.

gas•tric

gas•trin
plasma g.
serum g.

gas•tri•no•ma

gas•trit•ic

gas•tri•tis
antral g.
antrum g.
atrophic g.
atrophic-hyperplastic g.
catarrhal g.
chemical g.
chronic cystic g.
chronic follicular g.
cirrhotic g.
corrosive g.
eosinophilic g.
erosive g.
exfoliative g.
follicular g.
giant hypertrophic g.
hemorrhagic g.
hypertrophic g.

gas•tri•tis *(continued)*
phlegmonous g.
polypous g.
pseudomembranous g.
radiation g.
stress g.
superficial g.
toxic g.
zonal g.

gas•tro•ad•e•ni•tis

gas•tro•ady•nam•ic

gas•tro•anas•to•mo•sis

gas•tro•cam•era

gas•tro•cele

gas•tro•col•ic

gas•tro•co•li•tis

gas•tro•co•los•to•my

gas•tro•co•lot•o•my

gas•tro•cu•ta•ne•ous

gas•tro•di•a•phane

gas•tro•di•aph•a•nos•co•py

gas•tro•di•aph•a•ny

Gas•tro•dis•coi•des
G. hominis

gas•tro•du•o•de•nal

gas•tro•du•o•de•nec•to•my

gas•tro•du•o•de•ni•tis

gas•tro•du•o•de•nos•co•py

gas•tro•du•o•de•nos•to•my

gas•tro•dyn•ia

gas•tro•en•ter•al•gia

gas•tro•en•ter•ic

gas•tro•en•ter•i•tis
acute infectious g.
bacterial g.
eosinophilic g.

gas•tro•en•ter•i•tis *(continued)*
  viral g.

gas•tro•en•tero•anas•to•mo•sis

gas•tro•en•tero•co•li•tis

gas•tro•en•tero•co•los•to•my

gas•tro•ent•er•ol•o•gist

gas•tro•en•ter•ol•o•gy
  geriatric g.
  pediatric g.

gas•tro•en•ter•op•a•thy
  allergic g.

gas•tro•en•tero•plas•ty

gas•tro•en•ter•os•to•my
  short-loop retrocolic g.

gas•tro•en•ter•ot•o•my

gas•tro•ep•i•plo•ic

gas•tro•esoph•a•ge•al

gas•tro•esoph•a•gi•tis

gas•tro•esoph•a•gos•to•my

gas•tro•fi•ber•scope

gas•tro•gas•tros•to•my

gas•tro•gen•ic

Gas•tro•graf•in

gas•tro•graph

gas•tro•he•pat•ic

gas•tro•hep•a•ti•tis

gas•tro•il•e•ac

gas•tro•il•e•itis

gas•tro•il•e•os•to•my

gas•tro•in•tes•ti•nal

Gas•tro•in•tes•ti•nal Tu•mor Stu•dy Group

gas•tro•je•ju•no•col•ic

gas•tro•je•ju•no•esoph•a•gos•to•my

gas•tro•je•ju•nos•to•my
  Hofmeister anticolic g.

gas•tro•ki•neso•graph

gas•tro•lith

gas•tro•li•thi•a•sis

gas•trol•o•gist

gas•trol•o•gy

gas•trol•y•sis

Gas•tro•lyte

gas•tro•ma•la•cia

gas•tro•meg•a•ly

gas•tro•my•co•sis

gas•tro•my•ot•o•my

gas•tro•myx•or•rhea

gas•tro•pan•cre•a•ti•tis

gas•tro•pa•ral•y•sis

gas•tro•pa•re•sis

gas•tro•pa•ri•e•tal

gas•tro•path•ic

gas•trop•a•thy
  congestive g.

gas•tro•peri•odyn•ia

gas•tro•peri•to•ni•tis

gas•tro•pexy
  Hill posterior g.

gas•tro•pho•tog•ra•phy

gas•tro•phren•ic

gas•tro•phthis•is

gas•tro•plas•ty
  vertical banded g.

gas•tro•ple•gia

gas•tro•pli•ca•tion

gas•tro•pro•tec•tion
adaptive g.

gas•tro•py•lo•rec•to•my

gas•tro•py•lor•ic

gas•tror•rha•gia

gas•tror•rha•phy

gas•tror•rhea

gas•tror•rhex•is

gas•tro•scope
ACMI g.
Benedict g.
Cameron flexible g.
Chevalier Jackson g.
Eder g.
Eder-Chamberlin g.
Eder-Hufford g.
Eder-Palmer g.
Ellsner g.
fiberoptic g.
Herman-Taylor g.
Housset-Debray g.
Janeway g.
Kelling g.
Machida FGS-ML II magnifying g.
Machida FGS-SML magnifying g.
Olympus GIF-HM magnifying g.
Olympus GIF-M magnifying g.
Schindler g.
Wolf-Schindler g.

gas•tro•scop•ic

gas•tros•co•py
Stamm-Senn g. (Billroth type)

gas•tro•se•lec•tive

gas•tro•sia
g. fungosa

gas•tro•sis

Gas•tro•spi•ril•lum
G. hominis

gas•tro•stax•is

gas•tro•ste•no•sis

gas•tros•to•la•vage

gas•tros•to•ma

gas•tros•to•my
Beck g.
Beck-Jianu g.
endoscopic g.
feeding g.
Glassman g.
Janeway g.
Janeway stapled g.
operative g.
percutaneous g.
Stamm g.
Witzel g.

gas•tro•suc•cor•rhea
digestive g.

gas•tro•tome

gas•trot•o•my

gas•tro•to•nom•e•ter

gas•tro•to•nom•e•try

gas•tro•tox•in

gas•tro•trop•ic

gas•tro•tym•pa•ni•tes

Gas•tro•zep•in

Gas-X

Gaud•er•er
Ponsky-G. technique

Gau•tier
G. classification (for extrahepatic bile duct atresia)

gauze
Iodoform g.
Oxycel cotton and dry g.
Vaseline g.

Ga•vard
G's muscle

Gav•in
G.-Miller intestinal forceps
G.-Miller tissue forceps

Ga•vis•con

Ga•vis•con-2

Gay
G's glands

GB
gallbladder

GBD
gallbladder disease

GBS
gastric bypass surgery

GD
gastroduodenal

GE
gastroenterostomy
gastric emptying
gastroenteritis
gastroenterology

Gee
G.-Herter-Heubner syndrome
G.-Thaysen disease

Gel•a•mal

Gel•foam
G. plug

Gel•pi
G. retractor

Gel•u•sil

Gé•ly
G's suture

Gen•a•lac

gene
DCC (deleted in colon carcinoma) g.

gene *(continued)*
MCC (mutated in colorectal cancer) g.

Gen•er•lac

geno•tox•ic

Gen•ta•cin

Gen•ta•fair

Gen•ta•mar

gen•ta•mi•cin

Gent•lax S

Gen•tle Na•ture

Geo•cil•lin

Ge•o•pen

GEP
gastroenteropancreatic

GER
gastroesophageal reflux

GERD
gastroesophageal reflux disease

Ger•lach
G's valve

GET
gastric emptying time

GET 1/2
gastric emptying half-time

GF
gastric fluid
gluten-free

Gf
gastric fluid

GFD
gluten-free diet

GI
gastrointestinal

GIA
gastrointestinal assistant

Gi•ar•dia
G. lamblia

gi•ar•di•a•sis

GIA (gastrointestinal anastomotic) sta•pler

GIF XQ10 up•per en•do•scope

Gil•bert
G's cholemia
G. cystic duct forceps
G's disease
G's sign
G. syndrome

Gil•les•by
Puestow-G. procedure

Gil•li•ard
Dumon-G. prosthesis pushing tube
Savary-G. dilator

Gil•man
G.-Abrams gastric tube

Gio-Gan

Gior•da•no
G's sphincter

GIP
gastric inhibitory polypeptide

GIS
gas in stomach
gastrointestinal system

GI series
gastrointestinal series

GIT
gastrointestinal tract

GITSG
Gastrointestinal Tumor Study Group

GJ
gastrojejunostomy

GK
galactokinase

gland
acid g's
aggregate g's
agminated g's
anal g's
g's of biliary mucosa
Brunner's g's
cardiac g's
circumanal g's
Cobelli's g's
duodenal g's
esophageal g's
fundic g's
fundus g's
Galeati's g's
gastric g's
gastric g's, proper
Gay's g's
hepatic g's
intermediate g's
intestinal g's
g's of large intestine
lenticular g's of stomach
g's of Lieberkühn
mucous g's of duodenum
oxyntic g's
peptic g's
pyloric g's
salivary g's
g's of small intestine
submandibular g.
submaxillary g.
Theile's g's

glan•du•la *pl.* glan•du•lae
glandulae circumanales
glandulae duodenales
glandulae esophageae
glandulae gastricae [propriae]
glandulae hepaticae
glandulae intestinales
glandulae mucosae biliosae
glandulae oesophageae
glandulae pyloricae

Glas•gow cri•te•ria (for severity of pancreatitis)

Glass•man
G. basket
G. brush
G. gastrostomy
G. non-crushing gastrointestinal clamp
McNealy-G. clamp

gli•a•din

Glis•son
G's capsule

glis•so•ni•tis

glob•u•lin
corticosteroid-binding g.

glo•bus *pl.* glo•bi
g. hystericus

glot•tis *pl.* glot•ti•des

glou-glou

glu•ca•gon

glu•ca•gon•o•ma

glu•co•cor•ti•coid

glu•co•ki•nase

glu•co•neo•gen•e•sis

glu•cose

glu•cose phos•pha•tase

glu•cose phos•pha•tase de•fi•cien•cy

glue
tissue g.

glu•ta•mate de•hy•dro•gen•ase

glu•ta•mine

γ-glu•ta•myl ami•no•trans•fer•ase

glu•ta•ral•de•hyde

glu•ta•thi•one

Glu•zin•ski
G's test

Gly•cate

glyc•er•in
mineral oil, g., and phenolphthalein

glyc•er•ol•phos•phate ac•yl•trans•fer•ase

gly•cine

gly•co•cho•late

gly•co•de•oxy•cho•late

gly•co•gen

gly•co•ge•no•sis

gly•co•lip•id

gly•col•y•sis

gly•co•pro•tein
biliary g.
GP2 g.

gly•co•pyr•ro•late

gly•cos•ami•no•gly•can

gly•co•sul•fa•tase

gly•co•syl•a•tion

gly•cyl•glu•ta•mine

gly•cyl•sar•co•sine

Gly•rol

Gly•sen•nid

GM
gastric mucosa

Gme•lin
Rosenbach-G. test

G-My•cin

GN
gram negative

Gold
G. deep surgery forceps

Gold•bach•er
G. anoscope
G. proctoscope

Gold•berg
Frykman-G. procedure

Gold•stein
G's hematemesis

Go•LYTELY

Gom•co um•bil•i•cal clamp

Gos•set
G. self-retaining appendectomy retractor

Gould
G. inverted mattress suture

Gou•let
G. retractor

GP
gram-positive

GPC
gastric parietal cell

gr +
gram positive

gr –
gram negative

graft
omental g's

Gra•ham
G. deep surgery scissors
G. scale (for drug-induced gastric mucosal damage)
G. test

Gram
G. stain

Grant
G. gallbladder retractor

gran•ule
Kretz's g's
perichromatin g's

gran•u•lo•ma *pl.* gran•u•lo•mas, gran•u•lo•ma•ta
eosinophilic g.
hepatic g.

gran•u•lo•ma *(continued)*
hepatic sarcoid g.
tuberculous g.

gran•u•lo•ma•to•sis
lipophagic intestinal g.

gran•zyme
g. B

Gra•ser
G's diverticulum

grasp•er
polyp g.

Gray
G. cystic duct forceps

Green
G. cystic duct forceps

green
indocyanine g.

Grey Tur•ner
G.T's sign

Grif•fith
G's point

Grif•fo•nia
G. simplicifolia

Grof
Jendrassik and G. method for bilirubin

Gron•dahl
G.-Finney operation

groove
anal intersphincteric g.
esophageal g.
innominate g's
intersphincteric g.
Liebermeister's g's
paracolic g.

Gross
G. disease
G. test

GRP
gastrin-releasing peptide

Gru•ber
G.-Landzert fossa
Meckel-G. syndrome

Gruen•tzig
G. balloon catheter

Gryn•feltt
G. hernia
G's triangle
triangle of G. and Lesgaft

GS
gallstone
Gardner syndrome

GSE
gluten-sensitive enteropathy

GU
gastric ulcer

gua•nyl•in

guide
Coons g.
Eisenberg torque g.
J g.
Lunderquist torque g.

guide *(continued)*
soft-tipped g.
stool color g.
Wilson torque g.

guide•wire
J-tipped g.
Lunderquist torque control g.
spring-tipped g.

gul•let

Günz•berg
G's test

Gus•sen•bau•er
G's suture

gut
blind g.

gut•ter
lateral g.
paracolic g's
pericolic g.

GV
gastric volume

H

HA
hepatic artery
hepatitis A
hyperalimentation

HAA
hepatitis-associated antigen

hab•it
bowel h.

hair•ball

Ha•ley's M-O

halo•al•kane

hal•o•thane

Hal•sted
H. anastomosis
H. hemostat
H. hernioplasty
H. interrupted mattress suture
H. interrupted quilt suture
H. method
H's operation
H. suture

ham•ar•to•ma
mesenchymal h.

ham•ar•to•ma•tous

Ham•el
H's test

Ham•il•ton
H. deep surgery forceps

Hamp•ton
H's line

Han•hart
Richner-H. syndrome

Ha•not
H's cirrhosis
H's disease

Ha•not *(continued)*
H's syndrome

HAP
high amplitude peristalsis

hap•to•cor•rin

har•dero•por•phy•ria

har•dero•por•phy•rin•o•gen

Har•ring•ton
H. forceps
H. retractor
H. splanchnic retractor
H.-Mayo scissors

Har•ris
H's band
H. tube
H. tube suction

Hart•mann
H's colostomy
emergent H's procedure
H's operation
H's pouch
H's procedure
H's solution

haus•tral

haus•trum *pl.* haus•tra
haustra coli

HAV
hepatitis A virus

Hay
H's test

Hayes
H. anterior resection clamp
H. colon clamp

Hays
H.-de Alameida gastric reservoir

HB
hepatitis B

HB_c
hepatitis B core (antigen)

HB_e
hepatitis B e (antigen)

HB_s
hepatitis B surface (antigen)

HB_cAb
antibody to the hepatitis B core antigen

HB_eAb
antibody to the hepatitis B e antigen

HB_sAb
antibody to the hepatitis B surface antigen

HB-Ag
hepatitis B antigen

HB_cAg
hepatitis B core antigen

HB_eAg
hepatitis B e antigen

HB_sAg
hepatitis B surface antigen

HbCV
hepatitis B conjugate vaccine

HBIG
hepatitis B immune globulin

HBV
hepatitis B virus

HC
high calorie

HCD
high carbohydrate diet

HCF
hypocaloric carbohydrate feeding

HCl
hydrochloric acid

HCLF
high carbohydrate, low fiber

HCS
hematocystic

HCV
hepatitis C virus

HD
hydatid disease

HDL
high-density lipoprotein

HDL_1
Lp(a) lipoprotein

HDL_2
high-density lipoprotein

HDL_3
high-density lipoprotein

HDL-C
HDL-cholesterol

HDLP
high-density lipoprotein

HDV
hepatitis D virus
human delta virus

HE
human enteric

H&E
hematoxylin and eosin (stain)

head
h. of pancreas

heal·ing
mucosal h.
ulcer h.

Hea•ly
H. GI forceps

Hea•ney
H. needle holder

heart•burn

He•gar
H. needle holder

Hei•den•hain
H's cells

Hei•ne•ke
H.-Mikulicz operation
H.-Mikulicz pyloroplasty
H.-Mikulicz strictureplasty

Heis•ter
H's fold
spiral valve of H.
H's valve

Hel•frick
H. anal retractor

He•li•co•bac•ter
H. pylori

Hel•ler
H's esophagomyotomy
H's myotomy
H's operation

hel•minth

hel•min•them•e•sis

hel•min•thi•a•sis

hel•min•thic

hel•min•thism

hel•min•thoid

Hel•ve•ti•us
ligaments of H.

hema•fe•cia

hem•an•gi•o•ma
capillary h.
cavernous h.
mixed h.
visceral h.

hem•a•tem•e•sis
Goldstein's h.

hem•a•tin

hem•a•to•bil•ia

hem•a•to•ce•lia

hem•a•to•che•zia

hem•a•to•ma *pl.* hem•a•tomas
duodenal h.
perianal h.

he•ma•to•peri•to•ne•um

he•ma•tox•y•lin

heme

heme oxy•gen•ase

Heme•Se•lect

hemi•can•a•lic•u•lus

hemi•co•lec•to•my
left h.
right h.

hemi•gas•trec•to•my

hemi•hep•a•tec•to•my

hemi•py•lor•ec•to•my

he•mo•bil•ia

Hem•oc•cult

Hem•oc•cult II

Hem•oc•cult SENSA

he•mo•cho•le•cyst

he•mo•cho•le•cys•ti•tis

he•mo•clip

he•mo•glo•bino•cho•lia

he•mo•peri•to•ne•um

he•mo•proc•tia

Hemo•Quant

he•mor•rhage
- gastrointestinal h.
- intra-abdominal h.
- pelvic h.
- peptic ulcer h.

he•mor•rhoid
- bluish h.
- combined h.
- external h.
- internal h.
- lingual h.
- mixed h.
- mucocutaneous h.
- prolapsed h.
- right posterior h.
- strangulated h.
- thrombosed h.
- ventral h.

he•mor•rhoi•dal

he•mor•rhoid•ec•to•my
- closed h.
- excisional h.
- laser h.
- modified Whitehead h.
- open h.
- radical h.
- submucosal h.

he•mo•sid•er•o•sis
- hepatic h.

he•mo•sta•sis
- endoscopic h.

he•mo•stat
- Crile h.
- Halsted h.
- Kelly h.
- mosquito h.

He•mo•vac

HEN
- home enteral nutrition

Hen•ning
- H's sign

He•noch
- H's purpura

He•noch *(continued)*
- H.-Schönlein purpura
- H.-Schönlein syndrome
- Schönlein-H. disease
- Schönlein-H. purpura
- Schönlein-H. syndrome

Hen•ry
- Cheatle-H. incision
- H. approach
- H. femoral hernia repair
- H. incision

Hen•sing
- H's fold
- H's ligament

HEP
- hepatic

he•pad•na•vi•rus

Hep•a•hy•drin

he•par
- h. adiposum
- h. lobatum

hep•a•rin

hep•a•tal•gia

hep•a•ta•tro•phia

hep•a•tat•ro•phy

hep•a•tec•to•mize

hep•a•tec•to•my

he•pat•ic

He•pat•ic-Aid he•pat•ic for•mu•la

he•pat•i•co•cho•lan•gio•je•ju•nos•to•my

he•pat•i•co•cho•led•o•chos•to•my

he•pat•i•co•do•chot•o•my

he•pat•i•co•du•o•de•nos•to•my

he•pat•i•co•en•ter•os•to•my

he•pat•i•co•gas•tros•to•my

he•pat•i•co•je•ju•nos•to•my

he•pat•i•co•li•thot•o•my

he•pat•i•co•litho•trip•sy

he•pat•i•cos•to•my

he•pat•i•cot•o•my

hep•a•tism

hep•a•tit•i•des

hep•a•ti•tis *pl.* hep•a•ti•ti•des
- h. A
- acute parenchymatous h.
- alcoholic h.
- amebic h.
- anicteric h.
- autoimmune h.
- autoimmune chronic active h.
- h. B
- h. C
- cholangiolitic h.
- cholangitic h.
- cholestatic h.
- cholestatic viral h.
- chronic h.
- chronic active h.
- chronic aggressive h.
- chronic interstitial h.
- chronic lobular h.
- chronic persisting h.
- cytomegaloviral h.
- delta h.
- drug-induced h.
- h. E
- enterically transmitted non-A, non-B h. (ET-NANB)
- epidemic h.
- fulminant h.
- fulminant viral h.
- granulomatous h.
- halothane-induced h.
- homologous serum h.
- icteric h.

hep•a•ti•tis *(continued)*
- idiopathic autoimmune chronic active h.
- infectious h.
- inoculation h.
- ischemic h.
- isoniazid-induced h.
- long-incubation h.
- lupoid h.
- MS-1 h.
- MS-2 h.
- non-A, non-B h.
- nonspecific h.
- periportal h.
- plasma cell h.
- portal h.
- post-transfusion h.
- post-transplantation h.
- serum h.
- short-incubation h.
- subacute h.
- toxic h.
- transfusion h.
- viral h.

hep•a•to•bil•i•ary

hep•a•to•cele

hep•a•to•cel•lu•lar

hep•a•to•cho•lan•ge•itis

hep•a•to•cho•lan•gio•du•o•de•nos•to•my

hep•a•to•cho•lan•gio•ent•er•os•to•my

hep•a•to•cho•lan•gio•gas•tros•to•my

hep•a•to•cho•lan•gi•os•to•my

hep•a•to•cho•lan•gi•tis

hep•a•to•cir•rho•sis

hep•a•to•col•ic

hep•a•to•cys•tic

hep·a·to·cyte
ground-glass h.
multinucleated h.
oxyphilic h.
pericentral h.
periportal h.

hep·a·to·du·o·de·nos·to·my

hep·at·odyn·ia

hep·a·to·dys·tro·phy

hep·a·to·en·ter·ic

hep·a·to·en·ter·os·to·my

hep·a·tof·u·gal

hep·a·to·gas·tric

hep·a·to·gen·ic

hep·a·tog·e·nous

hep·a·tog·ra·phy

hep·a·to·li·e·no·meg·a·ly

He·pat·o·lite

hep·a·to·lith

hep·a·to·li·thec·to·my

hep·a·to·li·thi·a·sis

hep·a·tol·o·gist

hep·a·tol·o·gy

hep·a·tol·y·sis

hep·a·to·lyt·ic

hep·a·to·ma·la·cia

hep·a·to·me·ga·lia

hep·a·to·meg·a·ly

hep·a·to·mel·a·no·sis

hep·a·tom·e·try

hep·a·to·path

hep·a·top·a·thy

hep·a·to·peri·to·ni·tis

hep·a·top·e·tal

hep·a·to·pexy

hep·a·to·phle·bi·tis

hep·a·to·por·tal

hep·a·tor·rha·phy

hep·a·tor·rhex·is

hep·a·tos·co·py

hep·a·to·so·le·no·trop·ic

hep·a·to·sple·no·meg·a·ly

hep·a·tos·to·my

hep·a·tot·o·my
transthoracic h.

hep·a·to·tox·ic

hep·a·to·tox·i·ci·ty

hep·a·to·tox·in

hep·a·to·trop·ic

hep·a·tox·ic

HEPES
N-2-hydroxyethylpiperazine-*N*-2-ethane sulfonic acid

Her·ing
canals of H.

Her·man
H.-Taylor gastroscope

her·nia
abdominal h.
acquired h.
h. adiposa
axial hiatal h.
Barth's h.
Béclard's h.
cecal h.
Cloquet's h.
Cooper's h.
crural h.
diaphragmatic h.
direct h.
diverticular h.
duodenojejunal h.

her•nia *(continued)*
encysted h.
epigastric h.
external h.
extrasaccular h.
fat h.
femoral h.
foraminal h.
gastroesophageal h.
Grynfeltt h.
Hesselbach's h.
Hey's h.
hiatal h.
hiatus h.
Holthouse's h.
incisional h.
indirect h.
infantile h.
inguinal h.
inguinocrural h.
inguinofemoral h.
inguinoproperitoneal h.
inguinosuperficial h.
intermuscular h.
internal h.
interparietal h.
intersigmoid h.
interstitial h.
intra-abdominal h.
intraperitoneal h.
irreducible h.
ischiatic h.
ischiorectal h.
Krönlein's h.
labial h.
Laugier's h.
levator h.
Littre's h.
lumbar h.
mesenteric h.
mesocolic h.
Morgagni's h.
oblique h.
obturator h.
omental h.
paraduodenal h.
paraesophageal h.
parahiatal h.

her•nia *(continued)*
paraileostomy h.
parasaccular h.
parietal h.
pectineal h.
perineal h.
peristomal h.
Petit's h.
prevascular h.
properitoneal h.
pudendal h.
retrocecal h.
retrograde h.
retroperitoneal h.
retrovascular h.
Richter's h.
Rieux's h.
Rokitansky's h.
rolling h.
saddlebag h.
sciatic h.
scrotal h.
Serafini's h.
sliding h.
sliding hiatal h.
spigelian h.
Treitz's h.
Velpeau's h.
ventral h.
W h.
Wutzer h.

her•nio•ap•pen•dec•to•my

her•nio•en•ter•ot•o•my

her•nio•lap•a•rot•o•my

her•ni•ol•o•gy

her•nio•plas•ty
Halsted h.

her•nio•punc•ture

her•ni•or•rha•phy
Anson-McVay femoral h.
Berkowitz-Bellis h.

her•ni•ot•o•my

her•pes•vi•rus

Her•ter
 Gee-H.-Heubner syndrome
 H's infantilism
 Heubner-H. disease

Hes•sel•bach
 H's hernia
 H's ligament

het•ero•chy•lia

het•ero•lith

het•ero•pan•cre•a•tism

het•ero•phy•di•a•sis

Het•er•oph•y•es

het•ero•phy•i•a•sis

het•ero•to•pia
 gastric h.

Heub•ner
 Gee-Herter-H. syndrome
 H.-Herter disease

hexa•chlo•ro•ben•zene

hexa•me•tho•ni•um

hexa•meth•yl•mel•amine

hexo•cyc•li•um

hexo•ki•nase

Hey
 H's hernia

HF
 high fat

HFD
 high fiber diet

HG
 high glucose

hi•a•tus
 h. femoralis
 patulous h.
 h. of Winslow

HIDA (hepato-iminodiacetic acid) scan

Hill
 H. posterior gastropexy
 H.-Ferguson rectal retractor
 H.-Ferguson retractor

Hil•ton
 H's white line

hi•lus *pl.* hi•li
 h. hepatis

Hirsch
 H. contraction

Hirsch•man
 Buie-H. anoscope
 H. anoscope
 H. hemorrhoidal forceps
 H. proctoscope
 H.-Martin proctoscope

Hir•scho•witz
 H. gastroduodenal fiberscope

Hirsch•sprung
 H's disease

His•ta•log

His•ta•log test

his•ta•mine

His•tan•til

his•ti•dine

His•to•plas•ma
 H. capsulatum

HIV
 human immunodeficiency virus

HMM
 hexamethylmelamine

Hmm
 hexamethylmelamine

HNPCC
 hereditary nonpolyposis colon cancer

Hoch•e•negg
    H's operation

Hoesch
    H. test

Hoff•mann
    H.-Steinberg gastric reservoir

Hof•meis•ter
    Colp-H. technique
    H. anastomosis
    H. anticolic gastrojejunostomy
    H.-Finsterer technique

hold•er
    Adson needle h.
    Brown needle h.
    Hegar needle h.
    Kilner needle h.
    Masson needle h.
    Mayo needle h.
    Sarot needle h.

Hol•lan•der
    H. test

Hol•ter Pe•di•at•ric Pump 903

Hol•ter Pe•di•at•ric Pump 907

Holt•house
    H's hernia

Ho•ma•pin

ho•mat•ro•pine

hook
    Adson dissecting h.
    Barr fistula h.
    crypt h.
    Dandy nerve h.
    Pratt crypt h.
    Pratt rectal h.
    Rosser crypt h.
    skin h.
    Stewart crypt h.
    Welch Allyn rectal h.

hook•worm
    American h.
    European h.
    New World h.
    Old World h.

Hoop•er
    H. deep surgery scissors

Horn
    H's sign

Hors•ley
    H. technique

hor•to•be•zoar

Hous•set
    H.-Debray gastroscope

Hous•ton
    H's valves

How•ship
    H.-Romberg sign

Hoyt
    H. deep surgery forceps

HP
    hyperplastic polyp

HPD
    hematoporphyrin derivative dye
    high protein diet
    home peritoneal dialysis

HpD
    hepatoporphyrin

HPLC
    high-performance liquid chromatography

HPN
    home parenteral nutrition

HPP
    human pancreatic polypeptide

HPVG
    hepatic portal venous gas

Hue•ter
H's maneuver

Huf•ford
Eder-H. gastroscope

Hun•i•cutt
H.-Lee gastric reservoir

Hunt
H. colostomy clamp
H.–Limo-Basto gastric reservoir

Hup•pert
H's test
H.-Cole test

Hurst
H's bougie
H. dilator

Hur•witz
H. intestinal clamp

Husch•ke
gastropancreatic ligaments of H.
H's ligaments

HV
hepatic vein

H and V
hemigastrectomy and vagotomy

Hy-Cal cal•o•rie sup•ple•ment

hy•draero•peri•to•ne•um

hy•dra•gogue

hy•dra•la•zine

Hy•drea

hy•drepi•gas•tri•um

hy•dro•ap•pen•dix

hy•dro•bil•i•ru•bin

hy•dro•cele
hernial h.

hy•dro•chlo•ric acid

hy•dro•cho•le•cys•tis

hy•dro•cho•le•re•sis

hy•dro•cho•le•ret•ic

Hy•dro•cil In•stant

hy•dro•cor•ti•sone
h. acetate

Hy•dro•cor•tone

hy•dro•gen aden•o•sine tri•phos•pha•tase

hy•dro•hep•a•to•sis

hy•drol•y•sis *pl.* hy•drol•y•ses

hy•dro•lyze

hy•dro•pan•cre•a•to•sis

hy•dro•pneu•mo•peri•to•ne•um

Hy•drox•a•cen

hy•droxy•chlo•ro•quine

N-2-hy•droxy•eth•yl•pi•per•a•zine-*N′*-2-eth•ane sul•fon•ic ac•id

hy•droxy•meth•yl•bi•lane

hy•droxy•pro•line

3β-hy•drox•y-Δ^5-ste•roid de•hy•dro•gen•ase

hy•droxy•urea

hy•droxy•zine

hy•me•no•lep•i•a•sis

Hy•me•nol•e•pis
H. diminuta
H. nana

hyo•de•oxy•cho•late

hyo•scine
h. butylbromide

hyo•scy•amine
  atropine, h., scopolamine, and phenobarbital
  h. and phenobarbital
  h. and scopolamine
  h., scopolamine, and phenobarbital

Hyo•so•phen

Hy•paque

hy•per•ab•sorp•tion

hy•per•ac•id•i•ty
  gastric h.

hy•per•al•i•men•ta•tion

hy•per•bil•i•ru•bin•emia
  congenital h.
  conjugated h.
  constitutional h.
  h. I
  neonatal h.
  unconjugated h.

hy•per•cal•ce•mia

hy•per•ca•thar•sis

hy•per•ca•thar•tic

hy•per•chlor•hy•dria

hy•per•cho•les•ter•ol•emia

hy•per•cho•les•ter•ol•ia

hy•per•cho•lia

hy•per•chy•lia

hy•per•em•e•sis

hy•per•emet•ic

hy•per•glob•u•lin•emia

hy•per•gly•ce•mia

hy•per•hy•dro•chlo•ria

hy•per•hy•dro•chlo•rid•ia

hy•per•lip•id•emia

hy•per•mo•til•i•ty

hy•per•pan•cre•or•rhea

hy•per•pep•sia

hy•per•pep•sin•ia

hy•per•peri•stal•sis

hy•per•pla•sia
  biliary epithelial h.
  Brunner's gland h.
  crypt h.
  focal nodular h. (FNH)
  goblet cell h.
  nodular lymphoid h.

hy•per•se•cre•tion
  gastric h.

hy•per•ten•sion
  portal h.
  splenoportal h.

hy•per•thy•roid•ism

hy•per•thy•rox•in•emia

hy•per•tro•phy
  Billroth h.
  crypt h.
  gastroduodenal h.

hy•per•ty•ro•sin•emia

hy•per•uri•ce•mia

hy•per•vo•le•mia

hy•po•al•bu•min•emia

hy•po•bil•i•ru•bin•emia

hy•po•chlor•hy•dria

hy•po•chy•lia

hy•po•gan•gli•o•no•sis

hy•po•gly•ce•mia
  alcohol-induced h.

hy•po•he•pat•ia

hy•po•hy•dro•chlo•ria

hy•po•ka•le•mia

hy•po•lac•ta•sia

hy•po•na•tre•mia

hy•po•pan•cre•a•tism

hy•po•pan•cre•or•rhea

hy•po•pep•sia

hy•po•pep•sin•ia

hy•po•peri•stal•sis

hy•po•phos•pha•te•mia

hy•po•pla•sia
    bile duct h.

hy•pox•emia

hy•pox•ia
    hepatic h.

Hyr•tl
    H's sphincter

Hy•zine-50

I

IAB
  intra-abdominal

IAS
  internal anal sphincter

IBB
  intestinal brush border

IBD
  inflammatory bowel disease

IBW
  ideal body weight

IC
  intracisternal
  irritable colon

ICA
  ileocolic anastomosis

ic•ter•ic

ic•ter•us
  i. gravis
  i. typhoides

ID
  intraduodenal

IDA
  iminodiacetic acid

ida•ru•bi•cin

IDST
  intraductal secretin test

IEL
  intraepithelial leukocyte

ifos•fa•mide

IFP
  inflammatory fibroid polyp

IG
  intragastric

IH
  inguinal hernia

IIBD
  idiopathic inflammatory bowel disease

IJ
  intrajejunal

IL
  ileum

ILDL
  intermediate low-density lipoprotein

il•e•ac

il•e•al

ile•ec•to•my

il•e•itis
  backwash i.
  distal i.
  regional i.
  terminal i.

il•eo•ce•cal

il•eo•ce•cos•to•my

il•eo•ce•cum

il•eo•col•ic

il•eo•co•li•tis
  tuberculous i.
  i. ulcerosa chronica

il•eo•co•lon•ic

il•eo•co•los•to•my
  end-loop i.

il•eo•co•lot•o•my

il•eo•ile•os•to•my

il•eo•proc•tos•to•my

il•eo•rec•tal

il•eo•rec•tos•to•my

il•e•or•rha•phy

il•eo•sig•moid

il•eo•sig•moi•dos•to•my

il•e•os•to•my
  Brooke i.
  diverting i.
  end i.
  end-loop i.
  loop i.
  mucosal grafted i.

il•e•ot•o•my

il•eo•trans•vers•os•to•my

il•e•um
  collapsed i.
  distal i.
  duplex i.

il•e•us
  adynamic i.
  dynamic i.
  gallstone i.
  hyperdynamic i.
  mechanical i.
  occlusive i.
  paralytic i.
  i. paralyticus
  spastic i.

Il•o•sone

Il•o•ty•cin

Il•o•zyme

Il•o•zyme pan•cre•at•ic en•zymes

imag•ing
  color Doppler i.
  color flow i.
  color flow Doppler i.
  Doppler color flow i.
  Doppler flow i.
  magnetic resonance i. (MRI)
  radionuclide i.
  technetium i.
  thallium i.
  ultrasound i.

IMED 430 en•ter•al feed•ing pump

imi•no•di•ace•tic ac•id

imi•pen•em
  i. and cilastatin

imip•ra•mine

Imm•ther

im•mu•no•glob•u•lin
  biliary i.

im•mu•no•re•ac•tiv•i•ty
  cholecystokinin-like i.

im•mu•no•scin•tig•ra•phy

im•mu•no•ther•a•py

im•mu•no•tox•in
  anti-TAP-72 i.

Imo•di•um

im•pac•tion
  fecal i.

im•pres•sio *pl.* im•pres•si•o•nes
  i. cardiaca hepatis
  i. colica hepatis
  i. duodenales hepatis
  i. esophagea hepatis
  i. gastrica hepatis
  i. oesophagea hepatis
  i. renalis hepatis
  i. suprarenalis hepatis

im•pres•sion
  cardiac i.
  cardiac i. of liver
  colic i. of liver
  duodenal i. of liver
  esophageal i. of liver
  gastric i.
  gastric i. of liver
  renal i. of liver
  suprarenal i. of liver

Im•u•ran

in•acid•i•ty

in•ci•sion
abdominothoracic i.
Battle's i.
Battle-Jalaguier-Kammerer i.
Bevan's i.
celiotomy i.
Cheatle-Henry i.
Chernez i.
curved transverse i.
Czerny-Kocher-Perthes i.
Deaver's i.
elliptical i.
epigastric i.
Fowler-Weir i.
Garlock's i.
gridiron i.
Henry i.
infraumbilical midline i.
Kehr's i.
Kocher's i.
lateral transverse abdominal i.
lateral upper abdominal transverse i.
left lower paramedian i.
left lower pararectus i.
left lower quadrant i.
left paramedian i.
left subcostal i.
left transrectus i.
left transverse i.
left upper quadrant i.
lower abdominal i.
lower midline i.
low transverse abdominal i.
L-shaped i.
McBurney's i.
McBurney muscle-splitting i.
median lower abdominal i.
median upper abdominal i.
midline i.
midline vertical i.
midrectus i.
oblique inguinal i.
paramedian i.

in•ci•sion *(continued)*
pararectus i.
Pfannenstiel's i.
radial i.
right lower quadrant i.
right midrectus muscle-retracting i.
right paramedian i.
right pararectus midabdominal scar-excising i.
right rectus i.
right subcostal i.
right upper paramedian i.
right upper quadrant i.
Rockey-Davis i.
Rockey-Davis modification of McBurney i.
Salmon backcut i.
Sanders i.
semicircular i.
semilunar i.
subcostal i.
thoracoabdominal i.
transrectus i.
transverse i.
transverse low abdominal i.
transverse midabdominal i.
transverse umbilical i.
T-shaped i.
upper abdominal i.
upper abdominal midline i.
upper abdominal transverse i.
Wangensteen's i.

in•ci•sion and drain•age

in•ci•su•ra *pl.* in•ci•su•rae
i. angularis gastris
i. angularis ventriculi
i. cardiaca gastris
i. cardiaca ventriculi
i. interlobaris hepatis
i. ligamenti teretis
i. pancreatis

in•ci•su•ra *(continued)*
i. umbilicalis

in•ci•sure
cardiac i. of stomach
umbilical i.

in•clu•sion
glycogen i.

in•com•pe•tence
ileocecal i.

in•con•ti•nence
anal i.
fecal i.
i. of the feces
rectal i.

in•con•ti•nen•tia
i. alvi

In•di•ana var•i•ant ga•lac•tos•emia

in•di•ges•tion
acid i.
fat i.
gastric i.
intestinal i.
sugar i.

in•dig•i•ta•tion

in•do•meth•a•cin

in•du•ra•tion
fibroid i.
granular i.

in•er•tia
colonic i.

in•fan•ti•lism
celiac i.
hepatic i.
Herter's i.
intestinal i.

in•farct
bile i.

in•farc•tion
intestinal i.
mesenteric i.

in•fec•tion
delta i.
HIV i.
opportunistic i.
parasitic i.

in•fil•tra•tion
fatty i.

in•flam•ma•tion

In•fu•morph

in•fu•sion
bolus i.
constant i.
gastrojet i.

In•galls
I. rectal injection cannula

in•hib•i•tor
H^+ pump i.
lipoxygenase i.
protease i.
wheat amylase i.

in•jec•tion
intravariceal i.
vasopressin i.

in•ju•ry
alcohol-induced gastric i.
bile salt i.
gastric i.
hepatocellular i.
intestinal i.
ischemia-reperfusion i.
NSAID-induced gastric i.
NSAID-induced intestinal i.
oxidative i.
radiation i.

in•sorp•tion

In•sta-Char

in•suf•fi•cien•cy
gastric i.
gastromotor i.
hepatic i.
ileocecal i.

in•suf•fi•cien•cy *(continued)*
pancreatic i.

in•suf•fla•tion

in•suf•fla•tor

in•su•la *pl.* in•su•lae
insulae of Peyer

in•su•lin

in•su•li•no•ma

in•take
caloric i.
food i.

in•teg•ri•ty
mucosal i.

in•ter•fer•on
i. alfa-2a
i. alfa-2b
i. alfa-n1
i. alfa-n3
i.-β (IFN-β)
beta i.
lymphoblastoid i.
recombinant leukocyte A i.

in•ter•lob•u•lar

In•ter•na•tion•al Os•to•my As•so•ci•a•tion (IOA)

intest
intestinal
intestine

in•tes•ti•nal

in•tes•tine
blind i.
empty i.
iced i.
jejunoileal i.
large i.
mesenterial i.
segmented i.
small i.
straight i.

in•tes•ti•no-in•tes•ti•nal

in•tes•ti•num *pl.* in•tes•ti•na
i. caecum
i. crassum
i. ileum
i. jejunum
i. rectum
i. tenue
i. tenue mesenteriale

in•tol•er•ance
dietary protein i.
glucose i.
hereditary fructose i.
lactose i.

in•tra-ap•pen•dic•u•lar

in•tra•cis•ter•nal

in•tra•col•ic

in•tra•du•o•de•nal

in•tra•gas•tric

in•tra•he•pat•ic

in•tra•in•tes•ti•nal

in•tra•lu•mi•nal

in•tra•mu•co•sal

in•tra•pan•cre•at•ic

in•tra•rec•tal

in•tro•duc•er
Nottingham Key-Med i.

in•tro•gas•tric

in•tro•i•tus *pl.* in•tro•i•tus
i. oesophagi

In•tron A

in•tro•sus•cep•tion

in•tu•ba•tion
endoscopic i.
enterocutaneous i.
gastric i.
gastrointestinal i.
intestinal i.
jejunal i.
transgastrostomy i.

in•tu•ba•tion *(continued)*
transstomal i.

in•tus•sus•cep•tion
agonic i.
ileocolic i.
postmortem i.
retrograde i.

in•tus•sus•cep•tum

in•tus•sus•cip•i•ens

in•vag•i•na•tion

in•va•sion
lymphatic i.
pseudocarcinomatous i.

in•vert•er
Mayo-Boldt appendix i.
Mayo-Kelly appendix i.

IOA
International Ostomy Association

io•ce•tam•ic acid

io•dip•amide

io•hex•ol

io•no•my•cin

io•pa•no•ic acid

IORT
intraoperative radiotherapy

IP
ileoproctostomy
inactivated pepsin
infusion pump
intraperitoneal

IPAA
ileal pouch–anal anastomosis

ipo•date
i. calcium
i. sodium

ipro•ni•a•zid

IPSID
lymphoproliferative small intestinal disease

IR
ileal resection
intrarenal

IRA
ileorectal anastomosis

iron
serum i.

ir•ri•ta•bil•i•ty
i. of the stomach

IS
ileal segment
immune serum

is•che•mia
intestinal i.

is•che•mic

Iso•cal HCN tube feed•ing for•mu•la

Iso•cal pro•tein and cal•o•rie sup•ple•ment

Iso•cal tube feed•ing for•mu•la

iso•en•zyme
carcinofetal i's
carcinoplacental i's

Iso•fi•ber tube feed•ing for•mu•la

iso•flu•rane

iso•leu•cine

iso•leu•cine:pep•tide his•ti•dine

Iso•mil for•mu•la

iso•ni•a•zid

iso•pro•pa•mide

iso•pro•te•re•nol

iso•sor•bide

iso•sor•bide *(continued)*
  i. dinitrate
  i. mononitrate

Isos•po•ra
  I. belli

Iso•tein tube feed•ing for•mu•la

Is•ra•el
  I. retractor

IV
  intravenous

Iva•lon su•ture

Ive•mark
  I's syndrome

Ives
  I. anoscope

IVH
  intravenous hyperalimentation

IVN
  intravenous nutrition

J

Ja•bou•lay
J. button

Jack•son
J's membrane
J's veil

Ja•cobs
J.-Palmer laparoscope

Jane•way
J. gastrostomy
J. stapled gastrostomy

Jap•a•nese dys•en•tery

Jass
J. staging (for rectal carcinoma)

jaun•dice
acholuric j.
breast milk j.
cholestatic j.
Crigler-Najjar j.
epidemic j.
Epping j.
hepatocellular j.
hepatogenic j.
hepatogenous j.
homologous serum j.
human serum j.
infectious j.
infective j.
latent j.
malignant j.
mechanical j.
nonhemolytic j.
nonhemolytic j., congenital
nonhemolytic j., congenital familial
nonhemolytic j., familial
obstructive j.
regurgitation j.
retention j.

Ja•vor•ski (Jaworski)
J's test

Ja•wor•ski
J. bodies
J's corpuscles

JD
jejunal diverticulitis

Jeg•hers
Peutz-J. polyp
Peutz-J. syndrome

je•ju•nal

je•ju•nec•to•my

je•ju•ni•tis
ulcerative j.

je•ju•no•ce•cos•to•my

je•ju•no•co•los•to•my

je•ju•no•il•e•al

je•ju•no•il•e•itis

je•ju•no•il•e•os•to•my

je•ju•no•je•ju•nos•to•my

je•ju•nor•rha•phy

je•ju•nos•to•my
endoscopic j.
feeding j.
needle-catheter j.
percutaneous endoscopic j.
Roux-en-Y j.
Witzel j.

je•ju•not•o•my

je•ju•num

Jen•dras•sik
J. and Grof method for bilirubin

Jeune
 J's syndrome

Jev•i•ty tube feed•ing for•mu•la

JI
 jejunoileal

Ji•a•nu
 Beck-J. gastrostomy

JIB
 jejunoileal bypass

John•son
 Dubin-J. syndrome
 J. esophagogastrostomy

Jon•nes•co
 fossa of J.

JP
 juvenile polyposis

JR-E (gastric cancer) cell

JR-St (gastric cancer) cell

JS
 jejunal segment

ju•gum *pl.* ju•ga

juice
 gastric j.
 intestinal j.
 pancreatic j.
 pure pancreatic j.

junc•tion
 anorectal j.
 cardioesophageal j.
 esophagogastric j.
 gap j.
 gastroesophageal j.
 ileocecal j.

Jung•hans
 Wolff-J. test

jux•ta•py•lor•ic

K

Ka•der
K's operation

kan•a•my•cin

Kane
K. umbilical clamp

Kan•ga•roo De•liv•ery Sys•tem

Kan•ga•roo 200 en•ter•al feed•ing pump

Kan•ga•roo 324 en•ter•al feed•ing pump

Kan•ga•roo 330 en•ter•al feed•ing pump

Kan•ga•roo Feed•ing Set

Kan•trex

kan•y•em•ba

Kao-Con

ka•o•lin
k.-pectate
k. and pectin
k., pectin, belladonna alkaloids, and opium
k., pectin, and paregoric

Ka•o•pec•tate

Kao-tin

Ka•pec•to•lin

Ka•po•si
K's sarcoma

Kapp
K.-Beck colon clamp

Ka•sai
K. classification (for extrahepatic bile duct atresia)
K. operation

Ka•shi•wa•do
K's test

Kas•low
K. plastic stomach irrigation tube

Kas•of

Ka•su•gai
K. classification (for chronic pancreatitis)

KATO-III (gastric cancer) cell

KC
Kupffer cells

K-C

Kef•lin IV

Kehr
K. incision
K's T-tube

Keith
K. needle

Kel•ling
K. gastroscope

Kel•logg's Cas•tor Oil

Kel•ly
K. clamp
K. hemostat
K. proctoscope
K. retractor
K. sigmoidoscope
K's speculum
K's sphincteroscope
K.-Murphy forceps
K.-Murphy forceps, curved
Mayo-K. appendix inverter

ke•lot•o•my

Ken•my•cin

Kent
K. deep surgery forceps

Ke•o•feed 500 en•ter•al feed•ing pump

Ke•o•feed 3000 en•ter•al feed•ing pump

Ke•o•feed II en•ter•al feed•ing pump

Ke•o•feed en•ter•ic feed•ing bag

Ke•o•feed II feed•ing tube

Kep•ler
  Robinson-K.-Power water test

Ke•pone

Kerck•ring
  circular folds of K.
  K's folds
  K's valves

Kerr
  Parker-K. chromic suture
  Parker-K. forceps

ke•to ac•id

ke•to•con•a•zole

ke•to•gen•e•sis

ke•tone

ke•to•sis
  alcohol-induced k.

ke•to•ti•fen

Key-Med-At•kin•son en•do•pros•the•sis

Kier•nan
  K's spaces

Kil•ner
  K. needle holder

Kin•berg
  K's test

Ki•ne•sed

kink•ing
  tube k.

Kirk•lin
  Carman-K. meniscus complex
  Carman-K. meniscus sign

Kle•ban•off
  K. common duct bougie
  K. gallstone scoop

Kleen•spec dis•pos•able spec•u•lum

Kleen•spec fi•ber•op•tic dis•pos•able sig•moido•scope

Klemme
  K. self-retaining appendectomy retractor

KMI 50 en•ter•al feed•ing pump

KMI 60 en•ter•al feed•ing pump

knife
  Bard-Parker k.
  deep k.
  skin k.

Koch•er
  Allen-K. clamp
  K. clamp
  K's dilatation ulcer
  K. forceps
  K. incision
  K. maneuver
  K's operation
  K. retractor

koch•er•iza•tion

Kohl•rausch
  K's folds
  K's valves

ko•ly•pep•tic

Kon•dre•mul

Kö•nig
  K's syndrome

Kon•syl

Korn•zweig
Bassen-K. disease

Korte
Luer-K. gallstone scoop

K-P

K-Pek

K-Phen-50

Kras•ke
K's operation
K. position
K. roll

K-*ras* on•co•gene

Kretz
K's granules

Krön•lein
K's hernia

Kru•ken•berg
K's tumor
K's veins

Kry•o•stik

K-tube

Ku•drox

Kun•kel
Bearn-K. syndrome
Bearn-K.-Slater syndrome
K's syndrome

Kupf•fer
K's cells

Ku•ra•cil

Ku-Zyme HP

Ku-Zyme HP pan•cre•at•ic en•zymes

L

L
liver

la•bi•um *pl.* la•bia
l. inferius valvulae coli
l. superius valvulae coli

lac•er•a•tion
Mallory-Weiss l.

Lact-Aid

lac•tase

lac•tate

lac•tate de•hy•dro•gen•ase

L-lac•tate de•hy•dro•gen•ase (LDH)

lac•ti•tol

Lac•to•bac•il•lus
L. acidophilus

lac•tose
l. intolerance

Lac•tu•lax

lac•tu•lose

Ladd
L's bands

Laën•nec
L's cirrhosis
L's disease

La•hey
L. aneurysm needle
L. gall duct forceps
L.-Babcock forceps

lake
bile l.

lam•i•na *pl.* lam•i•nae
l. muscularis mucosae coli
l. muscularis mucosae esophagi
l. muscularis mucosae gastris
l. muscularis mucosae intestini crassi
l. muscularis mucosae intestini recti
l. muscularis mucosae intestini tenuis
l. muscularis mucosae oesophagi
l. muscularis mucosae recti
l. muscularis mucosae ventriculi
l. propria
submucous l. of stomach
vascular l. of stomach

lam•in•in

Land•zert
Gruber-L. fossa
L's fossa

Lane
L's bands
L's disease
L. dissecting forceps
L. forceps
L. gastroenterostomy catheter
L. gastroenterostomy clamp
L's operation
L. tissue forceps

Lang
L. suture

Lan•gen•beck
L. retractor

lan•so•pra•zole

Lan•soÿl

Lanz
L's point

Lan•za
L. scale (for drug-induced gastric mucosal damage)
modified L. scale (for drug-induced gastric mucosal damage)

Lap
laparotomy

lap
laparotomy

lap•a•ro•cho•le•cys•tot•o•my

lap•a•ro•co•lec•to•my

lap•a•ro•co•los•to•my

lap•a•ro•co•lot•o•my

lap•a•ro•en•ter•os•to•my

lap•a•ro•en•ter•ot•o•my

lap•a•ro•gas•tros•co•py

lap•a•ro•gas•tros•to•my

lap•a•ro•gas•trot•o•my

lap•a•ro•hep•a•tot•o•my

lap•a•ro•il•e•ot•o•my

lap•a•ro•scope
0-degree forward optic l.
10-degree optic operating l.
50-degree foroblique l.
Jacobs-Palmer l.

lap•a•ros•co•py
double-puncture l.
flexible l.
single-puncture l.

lap•a•rot•o•my
exploratory l.

lap•a•ro•typh•lot•o•my

La•pi•né
Chassard-L. projection

La•Roque
L. herniorrhaphy incision
L. repair

Lar•ry
L. rectal director
L. rectal probe

lar•va *pl.* lar•vae
visceral l. migrans

la•ser
argon l.
CO_2 l.
Medilas Nd:YAG l.
Molectron Nd:YAG l.
Nd:YAG l.
Olympus Nd:YAG l.
YAG l.

la•ten•cy
pudendal nerve terminal motor l. (PNTML)

Latz•ko
L. technique

Lau•bry
L.-Soulle syndrome

lau•da•num

Lau•gier
L's hernia

law
Courvoisier's l.

Law•rence
L. deep surgery forceps
L. gastric reservoir

lax•a•tion

lax•a•tive
bulk-forming l.
contact l.
emollient l.
hyperosmotic l.
lubricant l.
saline l.
stimulant l.

Lax•i•nate 100

Lax•it

lay•er
- Bernard's glandular l.
- circular l. of muscular tunic of colon
- circular l. of muscular tunic of rectum
- circular l. of muscular tunic of small intestine
- circular l. of muscular tunic of stomach
- inferior l. of pelvic diaphragm
- longitudinal l. of muscular tunic of colon
- longitudinal l. of muscular tunic of rectum
- longitudinal l. of muscular tunic of small intestine
- longitudinal l. of muscular tunic of stomach
- parietal l. of pelvic fascia
- submucous l. of colon
- submucous l. of small intestine
- submucous l. of stomach
- subserous l. of peritoneum
- superior l. of pelvic diaphragm
- visceral l. of pelvic fascia
- Zeissel's l.

LCAT
- lecithin-cholesterol acyltransferase

L.C. car•bo•hy•drate mod•ule

LCFA
- long-chain fatty acid

LCT
- long-chain triglyceride

LD
- liver disease

LDL
- low-density lipoprotein

LDL-C
- low-density lipoprotein cholesterol

LDLP
- low-density lipoprotein

LDS
- ligating and dividing stapler

leak
- anastomotic l.

Leb•sche
- L. shears

lec•i•thin

lec•i•thin-cho•les•ter•ol ac•yl•trans•fer•ase (LCAT)

lec•tin

lec•ture•scope

Lee
- Hunicutt-L. gastric reservoir

leio•myo•ma

leio•myo•sar•co•ma

Leish•ma•nia
- *L. donovani*
- *L. donovani chagasi*
- *L. donovani donovani*
- *L. donovani infantum*

leish•ma•nia

leish•ma•ni•al

Lem•bert
- Albert-L. suture
- Czerny-L. suture
- L. suture
- L. suture, continuous
- L. suture, interrupted

le•mo•pa•ral•y•sis

le•mo•ste•no•sis

Lenn•hoff
- L's sign

Leon•ard
 L. deep surgery forceps

LES
 lower esophageal sphincter

Les•gaft
 L's space
 L's triangle
 triangle of Grynfeltt and L.

le•sion
 apple core l.
 bull's-eye l.
 Dieulafoy's l.
 Dukes' A l.
 Dukes' B l.
 Dukes' C l.
 florid duct l.
 obstructing l.
 pedunculated l.
 polypoid l.
 sessile l.
 skip l's
 target l.

Les•tid

leu•cine

leu•co•vo•rin

Leu•ker•an

leu•ko•cyte
 fecal l.
 intraepithelial l.
 polymorphonuclear l.

leu•ko•uro•bi•lin

lev•am•i•sole

Lev•ate

Le•Veen
 L. shunt

lev•el
 air-fluid l.

Le•vin
 L. duodenal tube
 L. tube

Le•vin *(continued)*
 L. tube aspiration

Lev•sin•ex

Lew•is
 L. classification (for vascular anomalies of the gastrointestinal tract)

Ley•den
 L's disease

LFD
 lactose-free diet
 low-fat diet

LFS
 liver function series

LGI
 lower gastrointestinal

LHL
 left hepatic lobe

LI
 lactose intolerance

Lib•rax

Lib•ri•tabs

Lib•ri•um

Li•dox

Li•dox•ide

Lie•ber•kühn
 L's ampulla
 crypts of L.
 L's follicles
 glands of L.

Lie•ber•man
 L. proctoscope
 L. sigmoidoscope

Lie•ber•meis•ter
 L's furrows
 L's grooves

li•en•ter•ic

li•en•tery

lig•a•ment
- anterior l. of colon
- Arantius' l.
- broad l. of liver
- Clado's l.
- l's of colon
- coronary l. of liver
- costocolic l.
- cysticoduodenal l.
- duodenohepatic l.
- duodenorenal l.
- falciform l.
- falciform l. of liver
- gastrocolic l.
- gastrohepatic l.
- gastrolienal l.
- gastropancreatic l's of Huschke
- gastrophrenic l.
- gastrosplenic l.
- l's of Helvetius
- Hensing's l.
- hepatic l's
- hepaticophrenic l.
- hepatocolic l.
- hepatocystocolic l.
- hepatoduodenal l.
- hepatogastric l.
- hepatogastroduodenal l.
- hepatorenal l.
- hepatoumbilical l.
- Hesselbach's l.
- Huschke's l's
- inguinal l., posterior
- inguinal l. of Blumberg
- interfoveolar l.
- lateral l. of colon
- lateral l's of liver
- left triangular l. of liver
- lienophrenic l.
- lienorenal l.
- mesocolic l. of colon
- phrenicocolic l.
- phrenicolienal l.
- phrenicosplenic l.
- phrenocolic l.

lig•a•ment *(continued)*
- pyloric l's
- right triangular l.
- right triangular l. of liver
- serous l.
- splenocolic l.
- splenogastric l.
- splenophrenic l.
- splenorenal l.
- suspensory l. of liver
- suspensory l. of spleen
- l. of Treitz
- triangular l. of liver, left
- triangular l. of liver, right
- Tuffier's inferior l.
- venous l. of liver

lig•a•men•tum *pl.* lig•a•men•ta
- l. coronarium hepatis
- l. duodenorenale
- l. falciforme hepatis
- l. gastrocolicum
- l. gastrolienale
- l. gastrophrenicum
- l. gastrosplenicum
- ligamenta hepatis
- l. hepatocolicum
- l. hepatoduodenale
- l. hepatogastricum
- l. hepatorenale
- l. interfoveolare
- l. interfoveolare [Hesselbachi]
- l. lienorenale
- l. phrenicocolicum
- l. phrenicolienale
- l. phrenicosplenicum
- ligamenta pylori
- l. serosum
- l. splenorenale
- l. teres
- l. teres hepatis
- l. triangulare dextrum hepatis
- l. triangulare sinistrum hepatis
- l. venosum
- l. venosum [Arantii]

li•ga•tion
band l.
Barron l.
bile duct l.
l. of hemorrhoids
hepatic artery l.
rubber band l.
variceal l.

lig•a•tor
Barron L.
McGivney hemorrhoidal l.

lig•a•ture
Brunner l. set
elastic l.

limb
defunctionalized l.

Li•mo-Bas•to
Hunt–L.-B. gastric reservoir

Lin•coln
L. deep surgery scissors

line
anocutaneous l.
anorectal l.
central intravenous l.
Conradi's l.
crypt l.
dentate l.
Hampton l.
Hilton's white l.
mesenteric l.
pectinate l.
white l. of pelvis
Z l.

lin•ea *pl.* lin•eae
l. alba
l. anocutanea
l. anorectalis
l. semilunaris

li•ni•tis
l. plastica

Lin•ton
L. shunt

lin•to•pride

lip
inferior l. of ileocecal valve
superior l. of ileocecal valve

Li•pan•cre•a•tin

lip•ase
gastric l.
hepatic l.

lip•id
biliary l.

Lip•io•dol

lipo•cyte

lipo•dys•tro•phia
l. intestinalis

lipo•dys•tro•phy
intestinal l.

lipo•fus•cin

lipo•gran•u•lo•ma
hepatic l.

li•pol•y•sis

li•po•ma

lipo•pha•gia
l. granulomatosis

lipo•pro•tein
low-density l. (LDL)
very-high-density l. (VHDL)
l. X

lipo•trop•ic

li•pot•ro•pism

li•pot•ro•py

lipo•vi•ta•min

Li•pox•ide

li•poxy•ge•nase

LIQ
  lower inner quadrant

Li•qui-Char

Li•quid-A

Li•qui-Doss

li•quor *pl.* li•quors, li•quo•res
  l. entericus
  l. gastricus
  l. pancreaticus

lis•ter•i•o•sis

li•thi•a•sis
  appendicular l.
  pancreatic l.

lith•i•um
  l. carbonate

litho•cho•late

litho•cho•lic acid

li•thol•y•sis

litho•trip•sy
  electrohydraulic l.
  extracorporeal shock wave l.
  mechanical l.

litho•trip•ter

litho•trip•tor
  American Endoscopy l.
  electromagnetic telepaque l.
  mechanical l.
  piezoelectric l.
  spark-gap l.
  Wilson-Cook l.

litho•trite
  rotary gallstone l.
  Rotolith l.

Lit•tre
  L's hernia

Lit•win
  L. angled scissors

Liv•a•da•tis
  L. circular myotomy

liv•er
  acute fatty l.
  albuminoid l.
  alcoholic fatty l.
  amyloid l.
  biliary cirrhotic l.
  brimstone l.
  cirrhotic l.
  degraded l.
  drug-induced fatty l.
  l. failure
  fatty l.
  foamy l.
  frosted l.
  hobnail l.
  icing l.
  infantile l.
  iron l.
  nutmeg l.
  pigmented l.
  polycystic l.
  sago l.
  stasis l.
  sugar-icing l.
  waxy l.

Liv•ing•ston
  L's triangle

Liv•ing•stone
  Procter-L. endoprosthesis

LLQ
  left lower quadrant

load
  bilirubin l.

lobe
  appendicular l.
  caudate l. of liver
  hepatic l's
  left l. of liver
  linguiform l.
  l's of liver
  l. of liver, left
  l. of liver, right
  quadrate l. of liver

lobe *(continued)*
Riedel's l.
right l. of liver
spigelian l.

lob•u•la•tion
portal l.

lob•ule
hepatic l's
l's of liver
l. of pancreas
portal l.

lob•u•lus *pl.* lob•u•li
lobuli hepatis
l. pancreatis

lo•bus *pl.* lo•bi
l. caudatus
l. caudatus [Spigeli]
lobi hepatis
l. hepatis dexter
l. hepatis sinister
l. insularis
l. medius prostatae
l. quadratus hepatis
l. spigelii

Lock•wood
L. intestinal forceps
L.-Allis tissue forceps

lo•cus *pl.* lo•ci, lo•ca
FAP l.

Lo•fen•a•lac for•mu•la

Lo•fene

Lo•gen

Lo•ma•nate

Lo•mine

Lo•mo•til

lo•mus•tine

Long•mire
L. and Beal gastric reservoir

Lo•nox

loop
Roux l.
sentinel l.
snare l.

lo•per•amide

LOQ
lower outer quadrant

Lord
L's dilatation

Los An•ge•les var•i•ant ga•lac•tos•emia

Lo•sec

Lo•so•tron Plus

loss
fecal nitrogen l.

Lo•theis•sen
L. femoral hernia repair

Lo-Trol

lov•a•sta•tin

Love•lace
L. forceps

Low•er
L. gall duct forceps

Low•si•um

lox•i•glu•mide

lox•ti•dine

LP
lipoprotein
low protein

Lp(a)
lipoprotein little A antigen

LPL
lipoprotein lipase

LQ
lower quadrant

LRQ
lower right quadrant

LS
  liver and spleen

LT
  labile toxin

Lud•wig
  L.-Dickson-MacDonald classification (for primary biliary cirrhosis)

Lu•er
  L. syringe
  L.-Korte gallstone scoop

Lu•er-Lok sy•ringe

Lu•gol
  L's solution

lum•bo•co•los•to•my

lum•bo•co•lot•o•my

lu•men *pl.* lu•mi•na
  anal l.
  bowel l.
  duct l.
  duodenal l.
  gastrointestinal l.
  gut l.
  intestinal l.
  rectal l.

Lu•mi•nal

Lun•der•quist
  L. torque control guidewire
  L. torque guide

Lundh
  L. meal
  L. test

LUOQ
  left upper outer quadrant

LUQ
  left upper quadrant

Lusch•ka
  L's crypts
  L's ducts
  L's fossa

Lüt•ken
  L's sphincter

ly•ase

lym•phad•e•ni•tis
  mesenteric l.

lym•phan•gi•ec•ta•sia
  intestinal l.

lym•phan•gi•ec•ta•sis

lym•phat•ic

lym•phen•ter•itis

lymph node

lym•pho•cyte
  crypt intraepithelial l.
  intraepithelial l.
  lamina propria l.
  T l's

lym•pho•ma
  gastric l.
  gastrointestinal l.
  Mediterranean l.
  non-Hodgkin's l's

Lynch
  L. syndrome (I and II)

Ly•pho•cin

ly•sine

ly•so•some
  hepatic l.

Ly•tren

M
mechlorethamine hydrochloride

Maa•lox

Mac•al•is•ter
valve of M.

Mc•Bur•ney
M. appendectomy retractor
M's incision
M. muscle-splitting incision
M's operation
M's point
M. retractor
M's sign
Rockey-Davis modification of M. incision

Mc•Cleery
Miller-M. anastomosis clamp

Mac•Don•ald
Dean-M. gastric resection clamp
M. dissector

Mac•don•ald
Ludwig-Dickson-M. classification (for primary biliary cirrhosis)
M's test

Mac•ew•en
M's operation

Mc•Giv•ney
M. hemorrhoidal ligator

Ma•chi•da FCS-ML II mag•ni•fy•ing co•lono•scope

Ma•chi•da FGS-ML II mag•ni•fy•ing gas•tro•scope

ma•chine
von Petz sewing m.

Mc•In•doe
M. long scissors

Mac•ken•zie
M's point

Mc•Ken•zie
M. clip applying forceps

Mac•Lean
M's test

Mc•Lean
M.-Ring feeding tube

Mc•Nealy
M.-Glassman clamp

mac•ro•am•yl•a•se•mia

mac•ro•co•lon

mac•ro•glob•u•lin
alpha m.

ma•cro•nod•ule
non-neoplastic m.

mac•ro•nu•tri•ent

mac•ro•phage
hepatic m.

mac•ro•sig•moid

Mac•ro•tec

mac•u•la *pl.* mac•u•lae
m. adherens
maculae albidae
maculae lacteae
maculae tendineae

Mc•Vay
Anson-M. femoral herniorrhaphy
M. repair

Mad•den
M. intestinal clamp

mag•al•drate
m. and simethicone

ma·gen·stras·se

Mag·na·cal pro·tein and cal·o·rie sup·ple·ment

Mag·na·gel

Mag·na·tril

mag·ne·sia
- alumina and m.
- alumina, m., and calcium carbonate
- alumina, m., and simethicone
- calcium carbonate and m.
- calcium carbonate, m., and simethicone
- magnesium trisilicate, alumina, and m.
- simethicone, alumina, calcium carbonate, and m.

mag·ne·si·um
- alumina and m. carbonate
- alumina and m. trisilicate
- alumina, m. trisilicate, and sodium bicarbonate
- calcium and m. carbonates
- m. carbonate and sodium bicarbonate
- m. citrate
- m. glucoheptonate
- m. hydroxide
- m. hydroxide and mineral oil
- m. oxide
- serum m.
- m. sulfate
- m. trisilicate, alumina, and magnesia

mag·ne·to·gas·tro·gram

mag·ne·tom·e·try

Mag-Ox 400

mal·ab·sorp·tion
- postgastrectomy m.

mal·as·sim·i·la·tion

Mal·a·tal

mal·di·ges·tion

Mal·e·cot
- M. catheter

mal·for·ma·tion
- arteriovenous m. (AVM)
- bile duct m.
- Dieulafoy's vascular m.
- gastric arteriovenous m.
- submucosal arterial m.

Mall
- space of M.

Mal·la·mint

Mal·lo·ry
- M's bodies
- M.-Weiss laceration
- M.-Weiss syndrome
- M.-Weiss tear

mal·nu·tri·tion

mal·on·di·al·de·hyde

Ma·lo·ney
- M. bougie
- M. dilator

mal·o·nyl co·en·zyme A

mal·ro·ta·tion

mal·tose

mal·to·tri·ose

malt soup ex·tract

Malt·su·pex

Maly
- M's test

ma·neu·ver
- Hueter's m.
- Kocher m.
- U-turn m.

man·ni·tol

man·nose

ma•nom•e•ter
external m.

ma•nom•e•try
ambulatory m.
anal m.
anorectal m.
balloon reflex m.
ERCP m.
esophageal m.
water-perfused m.

mano•vo•lu•met•ry
dynamic m.

MAO
maximum acid output

Ma•ox

Ma•quet biopsy table

Mar•blen

Ma•re•zine

mar•gin
dentate m.
distal mucosal m.
invasive m.
m. of pancreas, superior

mar•go *pl.* mar•gi•nes
m. anterior hepatis
m. anterior pancreatis
m. inferior hepatis
m. inferior pancreatis
m. posterior pancreatis
m. superior pancreatis

mark•er
biological m.
chemical m.
radiolucent particulate m.
radiopaque m.
tumor m.

mark•ing
red wale m.

Mar•lex mesh

Mar•lex pros•the•sis

Mar•lex screen

Mar•lex sheet

Mar•shall
M. U-stitch suture
M. U suture

Mar•tel
M's clamp

Mar•tin
Hirschman-M. proctoscope
M. forceps
M. needle
M's speculum
M. and Davy speculum

Mar•zine

MAS
multiple anal sphincterotomies

mass
appendiceal m.
appendix m.
intraluminal m.
polypoid m.

Mas•son
M. needle holder

ma•te•ri•al
contrast m.

Mat•hews
M. speculum

ma•trix *pl.* ma•tri•ces
extracellular m.
m. of liver

mat•u•ra•tion
m. of stoma

Max•er•an

Max•o•lon

May•dl
M's operation

Ma•yo
curved M. clamp
curved M. scissors
Harrington-M. scissors

Ma•yo *(continued)*
M. clamp
M. common duct probe
M. common duct scoop
M. cystic duct scoop
M. gallstone scoop
M. intestinal needle
M. needle
M. needle holder
M's operation
M. scissors
M. stand
M.-Adams self-retaining appendectomy retractor
M.-Boldt appendix inverter
M.-Kelly appendix inverter
M.-Noble dissecting scissors
M.-Robson gallstone scoop
Ratliff-M. gallstone forceps
straight M. scissors

may•tan•sine

Ma•zi•con

MB
methylene blue
microbiological assay

MCC
mutated in colorectal cancer

MCC (mutated in colorectal cancer) gene

MCFA
medium-chain fatty acid

Mc•Gaw/Nu•tri•pro en•ter•al feed•ing bag

MCT
medium-chain triglyceride

MD-50

MD-60

MD-76

MDA
methylenedianiline

MD-Gas•tro•view

meal
barium m.
Lundh m.
oral fatty m.
retention m.
small bowel m.
test m.

mec•amyl•amine

MeCCNU
semustine

MeCcnu
semustine

mech•lor•eth•amine
m. hydrochloride

Meck•el
M's diverticulum
M.-Gruber syndrome

Med•i•cut can•nu•la

Med•i•cut cath•e•ter

Med•i•cut nee•dle

Med•i•cut IV nee•dle

Me•di•las Nd:YAG la•ser

Me•di•lax

Me•dil•i•um

Medi-Tech bi•po•lar probe

Medi-Tech steer•able cath•e•ter

Med•i•ter•ra•nean lym•pho•ma

me•di•um *pl.* me•dia, me•di•ums
contrast m.

Med•oc-Ce•les•tin en•do•pros•the•sis

Med•o•va•tions feed•ing tube

Med•ra•lone

Med•rol

Meek•er
M. deep surgery forceps

Me•fox•in

mega•ce•cum

mega•cho•led•o•chus

mega•co•lon
acquired m.
acquired functional m.
acute m.
aganglionic m.
congenital m.
m. congenitum
idiopathic m.
toxic m.

mega•du•o•de•num

mega•esoph•a•gus

meg•a•lo•esoph•a•gus

meg•a•lo•gas•tria

meg•a•lo•he•pat•ia

mega•rec•tum

mega•sig•moid

mel•a•nem•e•sis

mel•a•no•ma
familial atypical multiple mole m.
malignant m.

mel•a•no•sis
m. coli

me•le•na
m. vera

me•le•nic

mel•pha•lan

Melt•zer
M's sign

mem•bra•na *pl.* mem•bra•nae
m. abdominis
m. mucosa vesicae felleae

mem•brane
abdominal m.
apical m.
atretic m.
basement m.
basolateral m.
brush-border m.
canalicular m.
cell m.
Jackson's m.
mucous m. of colon
mucous m. of esophagus
mucous m. of gallbladder
mucous m. of rectum
mucous m. of small intestine
mucous m. of stomach
pericolic m.
pericolonic m.
phrenoesophageal m.
prolapsed mucous m.
submucous m. of stomach

Mé•né•tri•er
M's disease

Men•ghi•ni
M. needle
M. technique

Men•kes
M. syndrome

men•thol

me•pen•zo•late

me•per•i•dine hy•dro•chlo•ride

Me•pro•lone

mer•cap•to•pu•rine

6-mer•cap•to•pu•rine

Mer•i•tene tube feed•ing for•mu•la

Mer•si•lene suture

MES
  mucosal electrosensitivity

me•sal•a•mine

me•sal•a•zine

mes•a•ra•ic

mes•en•chy•mo•ma
  malignant m.

mes•en•ter•ec•to•my

mes•en•ter•ic

mes•en•ter•i•o•lum
  m. appendicis vermiformis
  m. processus vermiformis

mes•en•ter•io•pexy

mes•en•ter•i•or•rha•phy

mes•en•ter•i•pli•ca•tion

mes•en•ter•itis
  retractile m.

mes•en•te•ri•um

mes•en•tery
  m. of ascending part of colon
  common m., dorsal
  m. of descending part of colon
  m. of rectum
  m. of sigmoid colon
  m. of transverse part of colon
  m. of vermiform appendix

mes•en•tor•rha•phy

mesh
  Marlex m.

meso•ap•pen•di•ci•tis

meso•ap•pen•dix

meso•bil•i•ru•bin

mes•o•bil•i•ru•bin•o•gen

meso•bil•i•vi•o•lin

meso•ce•cal

meso•ce•cum

meso•col•ic

meso•co•lon
  m. ascendens
  ascending m.
  m. descendens
  descending m.
  iliac m.
  left m.
  pelvic m.
  right m.
  sigmoid m.
  m. sigmoideum
  transverse m.
  m. transversum

meso•co•lo•pexy

meso•co•lo•pli•ca•tion

meso•cyst

meso•derm

meso•der•mal

meso•gas•tri•um
  dorsal m.
  ventral m.

meso•ile•um

meso•je•ju•num

meso-omen•tum

meso•pexy

meso•rec•tum

mes•or•rha•phy

meso•sig•moid

meso•sig•moi•di•tis

meso•sig•moido•pexy

meso•ste•ni•um

me•tab•o•lism
  carbohydrate m.
  drug m.

meta•du•o•den•um

met•a•gen•ic

Meta•gon•i•mus
M. yokogawai

meta•ic•ter•ic

Met•a•mu•cil

meta•pla•sia
ductular m.
gastric m.
intestinal m.
pseudopyloric m.

me•tas•ta•sis
hepatic m.
liver m.
synchronous m.

me•te•or•ism

meth•a•cy•cline

meth•ane

meth•an•the•line

met•he•mo•glo•bin•emia

meth•i•cil•lin

meth•im•a•zole

me•thi•o•nine

meth•od
Brown's m.
diazo m. for bilirubin
Halsted m.
Jendrassik and Groff m. for bilirubin
Murphy m.
Rehfuss' m.
Siffert m.
Sippy m.
sucrose-gap m.

meth•o•trex•ate

meth•oxy•flu•rane

meth•sco•pol•amine

meth•yl CCNU

meth•yl•cel•lu•lose

meth•yl•ene•di•an•i•line

N-meth•yl•for•ma•mide

meth•yl-GAG

meth•yl•gly•ox•al *bis* gua•nyl•hy•dra•zone (MGBG)

meth•yl•pred•nis•o•lone
m. acetate

Me•ti•zol

met•o•clo•pra•mide

met•o•prine

Met•ric 21

Met•ro I.V.

me•tro•ni•da•zole

Mett
M's test

Met•zen•baum
M. forceps
M. scissors

Mey•en•burg
M's complexes

Mez•lin

mez•lo•cil•lin

MGBG
4-methoxydaunorubicin

MHN
massive hepatic necrosis

Mi-Acid

Mi•chel
M. clip

Mi•chi•gan in•tes•ti•nal for•ceps

mi•cro•body
hepatic m's

mi•cro•co•lon

mi•cro•elec•trode

mi•cro•fil•a•ment
hepatic m's

mi•cro•gall•blad•der

mi•cro•gas•tria

mi•cro•gran•u•lo•ma

mi•cro•ham•ar•to•ma

mi•cro•he•pat•ia

Mi•cro•lip•id fat mod•ule

mi•cro•nu•tri•ent

mi•cro•some

mi•cro•sphero•lith

Mi•cro•spor•i•da

mi•cro•spor•i•dan

mi•cro•spo•rid•i•an

mi•cro•spo•rid•i•o•sis

mi•cro•trans•du•cer

mi•cro•tu•bule
  hepatic m's

mi•cro•vil•lus *pl.* mi•cro•vil•li

mid•az•o•lam

mi•graine
  abdominal m.

Mik•u•licz
  Heineke-M. operation
  Heineke-M. pyloroplasty
  Heineke-M. strictureplasty
  M. clamp
  M. colostomy
  M's operation
  M. technique

Miles
  M. operation

milk
  acidophilus m.
  Bulgarian m.
  bulgaricus m.

Mil•ki•nol

Mil•ler
  Abbott-M. tube
  Cameron-M. electrocoagulation unit
  Cameron-M. monopolar electrode
  Cameron-M. suction-coagulator
  Gavin-M. intestinal forceps
  Gavin-M. tissue forceps
  M. double-end retractor
  M. rectal operating scissors
  M. rectal tube
  M.-Abbott double-lumen tube
  M.-Abbott intestinal tube
  M.-Abbott tube
  McCleery-M. anastomosis clamp
  Savary-M. scale (for esophagitis)

Mil•ner
  M. needle

min•er•al oil
  magnesium hydroxide and m.o.

mini-sto•ma

Mini•tec

Mi•no•cin

mi•no•cy•cline

Min•tox

Min•tox Plus

mi•ra•cid•i•um *pl.* mi•ra•cid•ia

Mi•riz•zi
  M. syndrome

mis•er•e•re mei

mi•so•pros•tol

mith•ra•my•cin

mi•to•gua•zone

mi•to•lac•tol

mi•to•my•cin
  m. C

mi•to•xan•trone

Mi•tro•lan

Mix•ter
  M. clamp
  M. common duct dilating probe
  M. forceps
  Paul-M. tube
  Thorek-M. gallbladder forceps

MM
  mucous membranes
  muscularis mucosa

mm
  mucous membrane

Mmc
  mitomycin C

MMC C
  mitomycin C

Mmc C
  mitomycin C

mm Hg
  millimeters of mercury

MO
  mineral oil

Mo•be•nol

mo•bi•li•za•tion
  rectal m.

Moc•tan•in

Mo•dane

Mo•du•cal car•bo•hy•drate mod•ule

mod•ule
  carbohydrate m.
  Casec protein m.

mod•ule *(continued)*
  fat m.
  L.C. carbohydrate m.
  Microlipid fat m.
  mineral m.
  Moducal carbohydrate m.
  Nutrisource Amino Acids protein m.
  Nutrisource Amino Acids-High BC protein m.
  Nutrisource carbohydrate m.
  Nutrisource Lipid-LCT fat m.
  Nutrisource Lipid-MCT fat m.
  P.C. carbohydrate m.
  Polycose carbohydrate m.
  Pro-Mix protein m.
  ProMax protein m.
  ProMod protein m.
  Propac protein m.
  protein m.
  Sumacal carbohydrate m.
  vitamin m.

Mohr
  M's test

Mo•la•toc

Mo•lec•tron Nd:YAG la•ser

mo•lyb•den•um

mon•i•tor•ing
  ambulatory m.
  pH m.

mono•amine ox•i•dase

mono•chlor•a•mine

mono•glyc•er•ide

mono•oc•ta•no•in

mono•sac•cha•ride

Mon•ta•gue
  M. proctoscope
  M. sigmoidoscope

Mont•gom•ery
M. strap
M. tape

Moon
Ferguson-M. rectal retractor

Moore
M. classification (for vascular anomalies of the gastrointestinal tract)
M. gallbladder spoon
M. gallstone scoop

MOPP
mechlorethamine, vincristine, procarbazine, and prednisone

Mo•re•no
M. gastroenterostomy clamp

Mor•gag•ni
columns of M.
crypt of M.
frenum of M.
M's hernia
M's valves
semilunar valves of M.
sinus of M.

Mo•ro•ney
State-M. gastric reservoir

mor•phine

Mor•phi•tec

Mor•ris
M. retractor

Mor•ri•son
Verner-M. syndrome

M.O.S.

Mosch•co•witz
M's operation

M.O.S.-S.R.

mo•til•in

mo•til•i•ty
anorectal m.
biliary m.
colonic m.
esophageal m.
gallbladder m.
gastric m.
GI m.
intestinal m.

Mo•til•i•um

Mo•to•fen

Mott
Parker-M. retractor

Moul•tier
M. contraction

mound
ulcer m.

mouse
peritoneal m.

mouth
Ceylon sore m.

move•ment
pendular m.
segmentation m.
vermicular m's

mox•a•lac•tam

Mox•am

Moy•ni•han
M. artery forceps
M. clamp
M. gall duct forceps
M. gallbladder forceps
M. gallstone probe
M. gallstone scoop
M. skin forceps
M. technique
M's test

MP
mercaptopurine

6-MP
6-mercaptopurine

Mp
 6-mercaptopurine

6-Mp
 6-mercaptopurine

MPI Py•ro•phos•phate

M S Con•tin

MSIR

MSUD for•mu•la

MUC
 mucosal ulcerative colitis

mu•cil•loid
 psyllium hydrophilic m. and carboxymethylcellulose
 psyllium hydrophilic m. and senna
 psyllium hydrophilic m. and sennosides

mu•cin

mu•co•co•li•tis

mu•co•en•ter•itis

mu•co•pro•tein

Mu•cor
 M. racemosus

mu•cor•my•co•sis

mu•co•sa
 cobblestone m.
 colonic m.
 esophageal m.
 gallbladder m.
 gastric m.
 intestinal m.
 muscularis mucosae
 nodular m.
 oxyntic m.
 pouch m.
 prolapsed m.
 rectal m.
 shaggy m.

mu•cus
 gastric m.

Muer
 M. anoscope

Mul•ti•pax

MUP
 motor unit potential

Mur•phy
 Barrett-M. intestinal thumb forceps
 Kelly-M. forceps
 M's button
 M. drip
 M. intestinal needle
 M. method
 M. punch
 M. retractor
 M. sign
 M's test
 sonographic M's sign

mus•cle
 bronchoesophageal m.
 circular m.
 circular smooth m.
 colonic smooth m.
 esophageal smooth m.
 gallbladder smooth m.
 gastric smooth m.
 Gavard's m.
 gracilis m.
 iliococcygeal m.
 iliococcygeus m.
 interfoveolar m.
 intestinal smooth m.
 levator ani m.
 longitudinal m.
 longitudinal smooth m.
 lymphatic smooth m.
 Ochsner's m.
 Oddi's m.
 pubicoperitoneal m.
 pubococcygeal m.
 pubococcygeus m.
 pyloric sphincter m.

mus•cle *(continued)*
  rectus m's
  smooth m.
  sphincter m. of anus, external
  sphincter m. of anus, internal
  sphincter m. of bile duct
  sphincter m. of hepatopancreatic ampulla
  sphincter m. of pylorus
  suspensory m. of duodenum
  m. of Treitz

mus•cu•la•ris
  m. mucosae
  m. propria

mus•cu•lus *pl.* mus•cu•li
  m. bronchoesophageus
  m. sphincter ampullae hepatopancreaticae
  m. sphincter ani externus
  m. sphincter ani internus
  m. sphincter ductus choledochi
  m. suspensorius duodeni

MUST
  mechlorethamine hydrochloride (Mustargen)

Must
  mechlorethamine hydrochloride (Mustargen)

Mus•tar•gen

mu•ta•gen

mu•ta•ge•nic•i•ty

Mu•ta•my•cin

mu•ta•tion

my•as•the•nia
  m. gastrica

My•co•bac•te•ri•um
  M. avium–intracellulare
  M. bovis
  M. tuberculosis

my•co•bac•te•ri•um *pl.* my•co•bac•te•ria

My-E

my•elo•per•ox•i•dase (MPO)

my•en•ter•ic

my•en•ter•on

My•ers
  M. and Fine test

My•gel

My•gel II

my•ia•sis
  intestinal m.

My•lan•ta

My•lan•ta-2 *(Canada)*

My•lan•ta-II *(U.S.)*

Myles
  M. hemorrhoidal clamp

My•li•con

My•li•us
  M. test

myo•fi•bro•blast

my•o•sin

my•ot•o•my
  Heller's m.
  Livadatis' circular m.

My•phen•tol

My•rhe
  Ruvalcaba-M.-Smith syndrome

myxo•glob•u•lo•sis

myx•or•rhea
  m. intestinalis

N

NABX
needle aspiration biopsy

Nach•las
N. gastrointestinal tube

Na•cle•rio
N's sign
V sign of N.

Naf•cil

naf•cil•lin

Naj•jar
Crigler-N. disease
Crigler-N. jaundice
Crigler-N. syndrome

Na•ka•ya•ma
N's test

Nall•pen

NANB
non-A, non-B (hepatitis)

na•prox•en

Nat•ur•a•cil

Na•ture's Rem•e•dy

nau•sea
n. epidemica

nau•se•ate

nau•seous

Na•vy sin•gle lay•er evert•ing anas•to•mo•sis

NBC
nasobiliary catheter

Nd:Yag (neodynium:yttrium-aluminum-garnet) la•ser

NE
needle electrode

Neb•cin

NEC
necrotizing enterocolitis

Ne•ca•tor
N. americanus

ne•ca•to•ri•a•sis

neck
n. of gallbladder
n. of pancreas

ne•cro•sis *pl.* ne•cro•ses
Balser's fatty n.
biliary n.
bridging n.
focal n.
hemorrhagic n.
hemorrhagic n. of liver
hyaline n.
massive hepatic n.
peripheral n.
piecemeal n.
piecemeal biliary n.
piecemeal hepatic n.
post-transplantation n.
sclerosing hyaline n.
subacute hepatic n.
submassive hepatic n.
zonal n.

nee•dle
aspirating n.
atraumatic n.
blunt point n.
Chiba n.
Childs-Phillips intestinal plication n.
cutting n.
Deschamps' ligature n.
eyeless n.
Ferguson n.
Frankfeldt hemorrhoidal n.
French eye n.
gastrointestinal n.
hernia n.

nee•dle *(continued)*
- Keith n.
- Lahey aneurysm n.
- Martin n.
- Mayo n.
- Mayo intestinal n.
- Medicut n.
- Medicut IV n.
- Menghini n.
- milliner's n.
- Milner n.
- Murphy intestinal n.
- regular intestinal n.
- reverse cutting n.
- sclerotherapy n.
- suture-release n.
- swaged n.
- taper n.
- taper point n.
- Tapercut n.
- Trocar n.
- Verres n.
- Vim-Silverman n.

nee•dle hold•er
- Crile-Wood n.h.
- Heaney n.h.
- Rogers n.h.
- Stratte n.h.

NEFA
- nonesterified fatty acids

Né•la•ton
- N's fold
- N's sphincter

Nel•son
- N. scissors
- Sprinz-N. syndrome

nem•a•to•cide

Nem•a•to•da

nem•a•tode

nem•a•to•di•a•sis

Nem•bu•tal

Nen•cki
- Sahli-N. test

neo•car•zi•no•stat•in

Neo-Cul•tol

Neo•lax

Neo•loid

Neo-Met•ric

neo•my•cin

neo•pla•sia

neo•plasm
- mucin-hypersecreting pancreatic n.

Neo•quess

neo•rec•tal

neo•rec•tum

neo•stig•mine

Neph•rox

nerve
- adrenergic n.
- cholinergic n's
- enteric n.
- hypogastric n.
- iliohypogastric n.
- non-adrenergic non-cholinergic n.
- peptidergic n.
- perineal n's
- phrenic n.
- splanchnic n's
- subcostal n.
- sympathetic n.
- vagal n.
- vagus n.

ner•vus *pl.* ner•vi
- n. hypogastricus
- n. hypogastricus dexter
- n. iliohypogastricus
- nervi perineales
- n. phrenicus
- n. subcostalis
- n. vagus

net•il•mi•cin

Net•ro•my•cin

Neu•bau•er
N. and Fischer's test

Neu•komm
N's test

neu•ro•fi•bro•ma

neu•ro•fil•a•ment

neu•ro•pep•tide
n. Y

Neu•tral•ca-S

ne•vus *pl.* ne•vi
hepatic n.

New•man
N. proctoscope

New•tri•tion tube feed•ing for•mu•la

NG
nasogastric

ni•a•cin

ni•a•cin•amide

ni•car•di•pine

nic•o•tine

ni•ge•ri•cin

Nis•sen
N. operation

nite•ca•pone

ni•tro•fu•ran•to•in

ni•tro•gen
blood urea n. (BUN)
n. mustards
urine urea n. (UUN)

ni•tro•phane

ni•tros•amine

N-ni•tro•so•meth•yl•urea

ni•za•ti•dine

NJ
nasojejunal

NJ (nasojejunal) feed•ing

No•ble
Mayo-N. dissecting scissors

node
abdominal lymph n's, parietal
abdominal lymph n's, visceral
anorectal lymph n's
appendicular lymph n's
celiac lymph n's
colic lymph n's
colic lymph n's, intermediate
colic lymph n's, left
colic lymph n's, middle
colic lymph n's, right
epigastric lymph n's, inferior
Ewald's n.
foraminal n.
gastric lymph n's, left
gastric lymph n's, right
gastroepiploic lymph n's, left
gastroepiploic lymph n's, right
gastro-omental lymph n's, left
gastro-omental lymph n's, right
hepatic lymph n's
ileocolic lymph n's
juxtaintestinal n's
lumbar lymph n's
lymph n.
mesenteric lymph n's, inferior
mesenteric lymph n's, superior
mesocolic lymph n's
pancreatic lymph n's

node *(continued)*
- pancreatic lymph n's, inferior
- pancreatic lymph n's, superior
- pancreaticoduodenal lymph n's, inferior
- pancreaticoduodenal lymph n's, superior
- paracolic lymph n's
- pararectal lymph n's
- precaval lymph n's
- prececal lymph n's
- pyloric lymph n's
- retrocecal lymph n's
- retropyloric lymph n's
- sentinel n.
- signal n.
- sigmoid n's
- splenic lymph n's
- subpyloric n's
- Troisier's n.
- Virchow's n.

nod•ule
- gastric lymphatic n.
- lymph n.
- lymphatic n's
- rectal lymphatic n.
- Sister Joseph's n.
- solitary lymphatic n's

nod•u•lus *pl.* nod•u•li
- n. lymphaticus
- noduli lymphatici aggregati [Peyeri]
- noduli lymphatici recti
- noduli lymphatici solitarii

no•dus *pl.* no•di
- n. foraminalis
- nodi juxta-intestinales
- n. lymphaticus
- nodi lymphatici abdominis viscerales
- nodi lymphatici anorectales
- nodi lymphatici appendiculares

no•dus *(continued)*
- nodi lymphatici coeliaci
- nodi lymphatici colici
- nodi lymphatici colici dextri
- nodi lymphatici colici medii
- nodi lymphatici colici sinistri
- nodi lymphatici epigastrici inferiores
- nodi lymphatici gastrici dextri
- nodi lymphatici gastrici sinistri
- nodi lymphatici gastroepiploici dextri
- nodi lymphatici gastroepiploici sinistri
- nodi lymphatici gastro-omentales dextri
- nodi lymphatici gastro-omentales sinistri
- nodi lymphatici hepatici
- nodi lymphatici ileocolici
- nodi lymphatici lienales
- nodi lymphatici lumbales
- nodi lymphatici mesenterici
- nodi lymphatici mesenterici inferiores
- nodi lymphatici mesenterici superiores
- nodi lymphatici pancreatici
- nodi lymphatici pancreatici inferiores
- nodi lymphatici pancreatici superiores
- nodi lymphatici pancreaticoduodenales inferiores
- nodi lymphatici pancreaticoduodenales superiores
- nodi lymphatici paracolici
- nodi lymphatici pararectales

no•dus *(continued)*
  nodi lymphatici precaecales
  nodi lymphatici precavales
  nodi lymphatici pylorici
  nodi lymphatici rectales superiores
  nodi lymphatici retrocaecales
  nodi lymphatici splenici
  nodi mesocolici
  nodi retropylorici
  nodi sigmoidei
  nodi subpylorici

Nol•va•dex

non•poly•po•sis

Nor•a•lac

nor•flox•a•cin

Nor-Mil

Nor•ox•in

Nor•panth

Nor•we•gian cho•le•sta•sis

Nor•wood
  N. rectal snare

notch
  angular n. of stomach
  cardiac n. of stomach
  n. of gallbladder
  gastric n.
  interlobar n.
  n. of ligamentum teres
  pancreatic n.
  transverse mucosal n.
  umbilical n.

Noth•na•gel
  N's bodies

Not•ting•ham-Key-Med in•tro•duc•er

No•va•mox•in

No•vo Am•pi•cil•lin

No•vo•bu•ta•mide

No•vo•chlo•ro•cap

No•vo•ci•met•ine

No•vo•hy•droxy•zin

No•vo•ni•da•zol

No•vo•pox•ide

No•vo•ryth•ro

No•vo•tet•ra

No•vo•tri•mel

No•vo•trip•tyn

NP
  nasopharyngeal
  nasopharynx

NPN
  nonprotein nitrogen

NPO
  L. nil per os (nothing by mouth)

NPS
  National Polyp Study

NPY
  neuropeptide Y

NRPRS
  nonrelaxing puborectalis syndrome

Nuck
  canal of N.

nu•cle•a•tion
  gallstone n.

nu•cleo•side
  tricyclic n. phosphate

5′-nu•cle•o•ti•dase

Nu•jol

NuLYTELY

Nur•soy for•mu•la

Nu-Tet•ra

Nu•tra•mi•gen for•mu•la

Nu•tra•pack tube feed•ing for•mu•la

Nu•tren 1.0 tube feed•ing for•mu•la

Nu•tren 1.5 tube feed•ing for•mu•la

Nu•tren 2.0 tube feed•ing for•mu•la

Nu•tri•pro EFS en•ter•al feed•ing pump

Nu•tri•source Ami•no Ac•ids-High BC pro•tein mod•ule

Nu•tri•source Ami•no Ac•ids pro•tein mod•ule

Nu•tri•source car•bo•hy•drate mod•ule

Nu•tri•source Lip•id-LCT fat mod•ule

Nu•tri•source Lip•id-MCT fat mod•ule

nu•tri•tion
- home enteral n. (HEN)
- home parenteral n. (HPN)
- home total parenteral n.
- modular enteral n.
- parenteral n.
- partial parenteral n. (PPN)
- supplemental parenteral n.
- total parenteral n.

Nut•tall
- N. liver retractor

N,V
- nausea, vomiting

N&V
- nausea and vomiting

NVD
- nausea, vomiting, and diarrhea

Ny•til•ax

O
obese
vincristine (Oncovin)

OA
Overeaters Anonymous

O'Beirne
O's sphincter
O's valve

obes•i•ty

ob•sti•pa•tion

ob•struc•tion
afferent loop o.
bile duct o.
biliary o.
colonic o.
common bile duct o.
efferent loop o.
false colonic o.
gastric o.
gastric outlet o.
intestinal o.
mechanical o.
obturation o.
outlet o.
pancreatic duct o.
papillary o.
portal vein o.
small bowel o.
stomal o.
strangulation o.

ob•tu•ra•tion

oc•clu•sion
enteromesenteric o.
mesenteric vascular o.

OCG
oral cholecystogram

Ochs•ner
O. clamp
O. forceps
O. gallbladder trocar

Ochs•ner *(continued)*
O. gallbladder tube
O's muscle
O's ring
O. spiral gallstone probe
Rochester-O. forceps

O'Con•nor
O.-O'Sullivan retractor

Oc•ta•mide

oc•tre•o•tide

Od•di
O's muscle
O's sphincter

od•di•tis

odyno•pha•gia

Ogil•vie
O's syndrome
O. technique

OH-urea
hydroxyurea

OI
opportunistic infection

oil
castor o.
corn o.
fish o.
131I-labeled iodized o.
medium-chain triglyceride (MCT) o.
mineral o.
mineral o. and cascara sagrada
mineral o., glycerin, and phenolphthalein
mineral o. and phenolphthalein

Old•field
O's syndrome

ol·i·go·pep·tide

ol·i·go·sac·cha·ride

ol·sal·a·zine so·di·um

Olym·pus/Alo·ka GF-EU1/ EU-M1 ul·tra·sound en·do·scop·ic sys·tem

Olym·pus CD-3L mono·po·lar probe

Olym·pus CF-HM mag·ni·fy·ing co·lono·scope

Olym·pus CF-ITS2 fi·ber·op·tic sig·moido·scope

Olym·pus CF-MB/LB co·lono·scope

Olym·pus CF-MB-M mag·ni·fy·ing co·lono·scope

Olym·pus CF-UHM mag·ni·fy·ing co·lono·scope

Olym·pus CPF-P10-S fi·ber·op·tic sig·moido·scope

Olym·pus GF-EU1 gas·tro·in·tes·ti·nal fi·ber·scope

Olym·pus GIF-D2 en·do·scope

Olym·pus GIF-D3 pan·en·do·scope

Olym·pus GIF-HM mag·ni·fy·ing gas·tro·scope

Olym·pus GIF-M mag·ni·fy·ing gas·tro·scope

Olym·pus GIF-P en·do·scope

Olym·pus GIF-2T en·do·scope

Olym·pus hot bi·op·sy for·ceps

Olym·pus Nd:YAG la·ser

Olym·pus nee·dle-knife pa·pil·lo·tome

Olym·pus OSF-60 fi·ber·op·tic sig·moido·scope

Olym·pus SIF-M mag·ni·fy·ing co·lono·scope

Olym·pus vi·deo co·lono·scope

Olym·pus vi·deo duo·de·no·scope

Olym·pus vi·deo en·do·scope

omen·ta

omen·tal

omen·tec·to·my

omen·ti·tis

omen·to·fix·a·tion

omen·to·pexy

omen·to·plas·ty

omen·tor·rha·phy

omen·tot·o·my

omen·to·vol·vu·lus

omen·tum *pl.* omen·ta
  colic o.
  gastrocolic o.
  gastrohepatic o.
  gastrosplenic o.
  greater o.
  lesser o.
  o. majus
  o. minus
  pancreaticosplenic o.
  splenogastric o.

omen·tum·ec·to·my

ome·pra·zole

Om·ni·paque

Om·ni·pen

om·pha·lo·mes·a·ra·ic

om·pha·lo·mes·en·ter·ic

on·co·gene
  c-*myc* o.
  K-*ras* o.

on•co•gene *(continued)*
  ras o.

On•co•vin

on•dan•se•tron

Oo•cho•ris•ti•ca

open•ing
  cardiac o.
  duodenal o. of stomach
  ileocecal o.
  o. to lesser sac of peritoneum
  pyloric o.
  o. of stomach, anterior
  o. of vermiform appendix

op•er•a•tion
  Amussat's o.
  Bassini's o.
  Battle's o.
  Belsey Mark IV o.
  Billroth's o.
  Brunschwig's o.
  Child o.
  Dennis and Varco o.
  Duhamel o.
  Finney's o.
  Frank's o.
  Fredet-Ramstedt o.
  Grondahl-Finney o.
  Halsted's o.
  Hartmann's o.
  Heineke-Mikulicz o.
  Heller's o.
  Hochenegg's o.
  Kader's o.
  Kasai o.
  Kocher's o.
  Kraske's o.
  Lane's o.
  McBurney's o.
  Macewen's o.
  Maydl's o.
  Mayo's o.
  Mikulicz's o.
  Miles' o.

op•er•a•tion *(continued)*
  Moschcowitz's o.
  Nissen o.
  palliative o.
  Polya's o.
  Ramstedt's o.
  Roux-en-Y o.
  Sawaguchi o.
  Soave o.
  Ssabanejew-Frank o.
  State o.
  Suruga o.
  Swenson's o.
  Tanner's o.
  Torek o.
  Waugh and Clagett o.
  Whipple's o.
  Whitehead's o.
  Witzel's o.
  Wölfler's o.

opis•thor•chi•a•sis

Opis•thor•chis
  O. sinensis
  O. viverrini

opi•um
  kaolin, pectin, belladonna alkaloids, and o.

Or•a•graf•in

Or•a•mide

Ora•trast

or•gan
  digestive o's

or•i•fice
  cardiac o.
  duodenal o. of stomach
  epiploic o.

or•i•gin
  ectodermal o.
  endodermal o.
  mesodermal o.

Or•i•nase

Or-Tyl

Os•ler
    O.-Walker-Rendu syndrome

Os•mo•glyn

os•mo•lar•i•ty

Os•mo•lite HN tube feed•ing for•mu•la

Os•mo•lite tube feed•ing for•mu•la

os•teo•dys•tro•phy
    hepatic o.

os•teo•sar•co•ma
    o. of colonic mesentery

os•ti•um *pl.* os•tia
    o. appendicis vermiformis
    o. cardiacum
    o. ileocaecale
    o. ileocecale
    o. pyloricum
    o. valvae ilealis

O'Sul•li•van
    O'Connor-O. retractor

Otis
    O. anoscope

Ot•ten•heim•er
    O. common duct dilator

OURQ
    outer upper right quadrant

out•put
    basal acid o. (BAO)
    maximum acid o. (MAO)
    peak acid o. (BAO)

over•growth
    bacterial o.

Ovol

ox•a•cil•lin

ox•i•dant

Oxy•cel
    O. cotton
    O. cotton and dry gauze

oxy•met•az•o•line

ox•yn•tic

oxy•phen•cy•cli•mine

oxy•phe•ni•sa•tin

oxy•phe•no•ni•um

oxy•phil

oxy•tet•ra•cy•cline

P

PABA (para-aminobenzoic acid) test

pace•mak•er
  gastric p.

pace•set•ter

pachy•peri•to•ni•tis

pack
  laparotomy p.
  Vaseline gauze p.

pack•ing
  iodoform gauze p.

pad
  ABD p.

pain
  abdominal p.
  epigastric p.
  gas p's
  griping p.
  hunger p.
  postprandial p.

PALA
  N-(phosphonacetyl)-L-aspartate

Pal•mer
  Eder-P. gastroscope
  Jacobs-P. laparoscope

PAM
  melphalan
  phenylalanine mustard

L-PAM
  melphalan

Pam
  melphalan

L-Pam
  melphalan

Pam•ine

Pan•coate

pan•co•lec•to•my

pan•cre•al•gia

pan•cre•as *pl.* pan•cre•a•ta
  aberrant p.
  p. accessorium
  accessory p.
  annular p.
  p. divisum
  lesser p.
  Willis' p.
  Winslow's p.

Pan•cre•ase pan•cre•at•ic en•zymes

pan•cre•a•stat•in

pan•cre•a•ta

pan•cre•a•tal•gia

pan•cre•a•tec•to•my

pan•cre•at•ic

pan•cre•at•i•co•du•o•de•nal

pan•cre•at•i•co•du•o•de•nec•to•my

pan•cre•at•i•co•du•o•de•nos•to•my

pan•cre•at•i•co•en•ter•os•to•my

pan•cre•at•i•co•gas•tros•to•my

pan•cre•at•i•co•je•ju•nos•to•my

pan•cre•at•ic phos•pho•lip•ase A_2

pan•cre•a•tin

pan•cre•a•ti•tis
  acute p.
  acute alcoholic p.
  acute hemorrhagic p.

pan·cre·a·ti·tis *(continued)*
- biliary p.
- calcereous p.
- centrilobar p.
- chronic p.
- chronic relapsing p.
- focal p.
- gallstone p.
- interstitial p.
- necrotizing p.
- perilobar p.
- purulent p.

pan·cre·a·to·du·o·de·nec·to·my

pan·cre·a·to·du·o·de·nos·to·my

pan·cre·a·to·en·ter·os·to·my

pan·cre·a·to·gen·ic

pan·cre·a·tog·e·nous

pan·cre·a·to·gram

pan·cre·a·to·graph·ic

pan·cre·a·tog·ra·phy

pan·cre·ato·lith

pan·cre·a·to·li·thec·to·my

pan·cre·a·to·li·thi·a·sis

pan·cre·a·to·li·thot·o·my

pan·cre·a·tol·y·sis

pan·cre·a·to·lyt·ic

pan·cre·at·o·my

pan·cre·a·tos·co·py
- peroral p.

pan·cre·a·tot·o·my

pan·cre·a·to·trop·ic

pan·cre·a·trop·ic

pan·cre·ec·to·my

pan·cre·li·pase

pan·creo·li·thot·o·my

pan·cre·ol·y·sis

pan·creo·lyt·ic

pan·creo·ther·a·py

pan·cre·o·trop·ic

Pan·da feed·ing tube

pan·en·do·scope
- fiberscopic p.
- Olympus GIF-D3 p.
- upper gastrointestinal p.

pan·en·dos·co·py
- lower p.

Pan·eth
- P's cells

pan·proc·to·co·lec·to·my

Pant·ing
- P. self-retaining abdominal retractor

pan·to·pra·zole

Pan·zer
- P. gallbladder scissors

PAO
- peak acid output

PAP
- pancreatitis-associated protein

Pa·pa·nic·o·laou
- P. stain

pa·pav·er·ine

pa·pil·la *pl.* pa·pil·lae
- bile p.
- duodenal p.
- duodenal p., major
- duodenal p., minor
- p. duodeni major
- p. duodeni minor
- p. duodeni [Santorini]
- hypertrophic p.
- hypertrophic anal p.

pa•pil•la *(continued)*
ileal p.
p. ilealis
p. ileocaecalis
ileocecal p.
major duodenal p.
minor duodenal p.
p. of Santorini
p. of Vater

pap•il•lo•ma•to•sis
biliary p.

pap•il•lo•sphinc•ter•ot•o•my

pap•il•lo•tome
Erlangen p.
Olympus needle-knife p.

pap•il•lot•o•my

para-ap•pen•di•ci•tis

para•cen•te•sis
abdominal p.

para•cen•tet•ic

para•co•li•tis

para•esoph•a•ge•al

para•he•pat•ic

para•hep•a•ti•tis

para•il•e•ost•o•my

para•pan•cre•at•ic

para•peri•to•ne•al

Par•a•pla•tin

para•proc•ti•tis

para•proc•ti•um

para•quat

para•rec•tal

para•si•nu•soi•dal

par•a•si•to•sis

para•typh•li•tis

par•e•gor•ic
kaolin, pectin, and p.

Par•e•pec•to•lin

par•epi•gas•tric

pa•ri•es *pl.* pa•ri•etes
p. anterior gastricus
p. anterior ventriculi
p. posterior gastricus
p. posterior ventriculi

Par•ker
Bard-P. blade
Bard-P. scissors
P. retractor
P. ribbon retractor
P.-Kerr chromic suture
P.-Kerr forceps
P.-Mott retractor

Par•kin•son
P's disease

par•o•mo•my•cin

pars *pl.* par•tes
p. abdominalis esophagi
p. abdominalis oesophagi
p. analis recti
p. anterior faciei diaphragmaticae hepatis
p. ascendens duodeni
p. cardiaca gastris
p. cardiaca ventriculi
p. cervicalis esophagi
p. cervicalis oesophagi
p. descendens duodeni
p. dextra faciei diaphragmaticae hepatis
p. exocrina pancreatis
p. horizontalis duodeni
p. inferior duodeni
p. posterior faciei diaphragmaticae hepatis
p. profunda musculi sphincteris ani externi
p. pylorica gastris
p. pylorica ventriculi
p. quadrata

pars *(continued)*
- p. subcutanea musculi sphincteris ani externi
- p. superficialis musculi sphincteris ani externi
- p. superior duodeni
- p. superior faciei diaphragmaticae hepatis
- p. thoracica esophagi
- p. thoracica oesophagi

part
- colic p. of omentum
- inferior p. of duodenum
- parietal p. of pelvic fascia
- subphrenic p. of esophagus
- visceral p. of pelvic fascia

par•ti•tion•ing
- gastric p.

pas•sage

Pa•tel•la
- P's disease

Pa•thi•lon

Path•o•cil

path•o•gen
- enteric p.

path•way
- cystathionine p.

pat•tern
- brush p.
- cobblestone p.
- edge p.
- fingerprint p.
- flocculation p.
- haustral p.
- herringbone p.
- hidebound p.
- rugal p.
- spike p.
- stepladder p.

Paul
- P.-Mixter tube

Pau•ly
- P's point

Payr
- P. clamp
- P's disease
- P. gastrointestinal clamp
- P. pylorus clamp
- P.-Strauss contraction

PBG
- porphobilinogen

PBX
- punch biopsy

PCBs
- polychlorinated biphenyls

P.C. car•bo•hy•drate mod•ule

PCE Dis•per•tab

PCI
- pneumatosis cystoides intestinalis

PCNU

PCPS
- peroral cholangiopancreatoscopy

PCS
- peroral cholangioscopy

PD
- potential difference

PE
- pharyngoesophageal

Pé•an
- P. artery forceps
- P. clamp
- P. forceps
- P. GI forceps
- P. grasping forceps
- Rochester-P. forceps

pec•ten *pl.* pec•ti•nes
- p. of anal canal
- p. analis

pec•te•ni•tis

pec•te•no•sis

pec•te•not•o•my

pec•tin
  kaolin and p.
  kaolin, p., belladonna alkaloids, and opium
  kaolin, p., and paregoric

Ped•i•a•lyte

Ped•i•a•my•cin

ped•i•cle
  hemorrhoidal p.
  lymphovascular p.

pe•dun•cu•lat•ed

PEG
  percutaneous endoscopic gastrostomy

pel•i•o•sis
  p. hepatis
  p. of liver

pel•vio•peri•to•ni•tis

pel•vi•peri•to•ni•tis

pel•vi•rec•tal

Pem•ber•ton
  P. anastomosis forceps
  P. sigmoid anastomosis clamp

Pen•brit•in

pen•cil
  cautery p.

Pen•globe

Pen•ning•ton
  P. clamp
  P. hemorrhoidal forceps

Pen•rose
  P. drain

pen•ta•gas•trin

Pen•tax FS-34A fi•ber•op•tic sig•moido•scope

Pen•ta•zine

pen•to•bar•bi•tal

pen•tose

Pep•cid

pep•sic

pep•sin

pep•sin•ia

pep•sin•if•er•ous

pep•sin•o•gen

Pep•ta•men tube feed•ing for•mu•la

Pep•tav•lon

pep•tic

pep•tide
  calcitonin gene–related p.
  gastric inhibitory p.
  gastrin-releasing p.
  glucose-dependent insulinotrophic p.
  vasoactive intestinal p. (VIP)
  p. YY

pep•tide his•ti•dine iso•leu•cine

pep•tide hy•dro•lase

Pep•ti-2000 tube feed•ing for•mu•la

Pep•to-Bis•mol

Pep•to Di•ar•rhea Con•trol

pep•to•gen•ic

pep•tog•e•nous

Pep•tol

Per•cy
  P. intestinal forceps
  P. tissue forceps
  P.-Wolfson retractor

Per•di•em

per•fo•ra•tion
    common bile duct p.
    esophageal p.
    free p.

per•fu•sion
    biliary p.

per•hex•i•line mal•e•ate

peri•am•pul•lary

peri•anal

peri•an•gio•cho•li•tis

peri•ap•pen•di•ci•tis

peri•ap•pen•dic•u•lar

peri•ce•cal

peri•ce•ci•tis

peri•cho•lan•gi•tis

peri•cho•le•cys•ti•tis
    gaseous p.

Peri-Co•lace

peri•co•lic

peri•co•li•tis
    p. dextra
    membranous p.
    p. sinistra

peri•co•lon•ic

peri•co•lon•itis

peri•di•ver•tic•u•li•tis

peri•duc•tal

peri•du•o•de•ni•tis

peri•en•ter•ic

peri•en•ter•itis

peri•esoph•a•ge•al

peri•esoph•a•gi•tis

peri•gas•tric

peri•gas•tri•tis

peri•he•pat•ic

peri•hep•a•ti•tis
    chlamydial p.
    chronic diffuse p.
    p. chronica hyperplastica
    gonococcal p.

peri•je•ju•ni•tis

peri•ne•um

peri•pan•cre•at•ic

peri•pan•cre•a•ti•tis

peri•pap•il•lary

peri•proc•tic

peri•proc•ti•tis

peri•py•lo•ric

peri•rec•tal

peri•rec•ti•tis

peri•sig•moid•itis

peri•stal•sis
    mass p.
    retrograde p.
    reversed p.

peri•stal•tic

Peritf
    peritoneal fluid

peri•to•ne•al

peri•to•ne•al•gia

peri•to•ne•al•iza•tion

peri•to•ne•al•ize

peri•to•neo•cen•te•sis

peri•to•neo•cly•sis

peri•to•neo•mus•cu•lar

peri•to•ne•op•a•thy

peri•to•neo•plas•ty

peri•to•neo•tome

peri•to•ne•um
    abdominal p.

peri•to•ne•um *(continued)*
intestinal p.
visceral p.
p. viscerale

peri•to•ni•tis
adhesive p.
bacterial p.
bile p.
biliary p.
chemical p.
p. chronica fibrosa encapsulans
circumscribed p.
p. deformans
diaphragmatic p.
diffuse p.
p. encapsulans
encysted p.
fecal p.
fibrocaseous p.
gas p.
general p.
hemorrhagic p.
localized p.
pelvic p.
perforative p.
plastic p.
purulent p.
septic p.
serous p.
silent p.
spontaneous bacterial p.
terminal p.
traumatic p.
tuberculous p.

peri•to•ni•za•tion

peri•to•nize

peri•typh•lic

peri•typh•li•tis
p. actinomycotica

Per•ma-Hand su•ture

per•me•a•bil•i•ty
capillary p.
intestinal p.

pe•rox•i•dase
intestinal p.

per•ox•i•da•tion
lipid p.

pe•rox•i•some
hepatic p's

Per•ry
P. bag

Per•thes
Czerny-Kocher-P. incision

Pe•tit
P's hernia

Pet•ro•gal•ar Plain

Peutz
P.-Jeghers polyp
P.-Jeghers syndrome

Pey•er
insulae of P.
P's patches

Pez•zer
P. catheter
P. drain

Pfan•nen•stiel
P's incision

Pfuhl
P's sign

PG
phosphatidylglycerol

PGI
prostacyclin

P-gly•co•pro•tein

pH (hydrogen ion concentration)
colonic pH
esophageal pH
gastric pH
intestinal pH

phar•ma•co•an•gi•og•ra•phy

pha•ryn•gos•to•my

phar•ynx

Pha•zyme

Phen•a•meth

Phen•a•zine

Phen•cen-50

Phen•er•gan

phe•net•i•din

phe•no•bar•bi•tal
- atropine and p.
- atropine, hyoscyamine, scopolamine, and p.
- belladonna and p.
- hyoscyamine and p.
- hyoscyamine, scopolamine, and p.

Phe•no•ject-50

Phe•no•lax

phe•nol•phthal•ein
- cascara sagrada and p.
- dehydrochloric acid, docusate, and p.
- docusate and p.
- mineral oil and p.
- mineral oil, glycerin, and p.

Phe•nol•phthal•ein Pet•ro•gal•ar

phe•nom•e•non *pl.* phe•nom•e•na
- walking stick p.

phen•yl•al•a•nine

phen•yl•bu•ta•zone

phen•y•to•in

PHI
- peptide histidine isoleucine

Phil•ips RT50 ra•dio•ther•a•py unit

Phil•lips
- Childs-P. intestinal plication needle
- P. rectal clamp

Phil•lips' Lax•Caps

Phil•lips' Mag•ne•sia Tab•lets

Phil•lips' Milk of Mag•ne•sia

phleb•ec•ta•sia

phleg•mon
- pancreatic p.

phlo•rhi•zin hy•dro•lase

phos•pha•ti•dyl•cho•line

phos•pha•ti•dyl•eth•a•nol•amine

phos•pha•ti•dyl•glyc•er•ol

phos•pha•ti•dyl•in•o•si•tol

phos•pho•ino•si•tide

phos•pho•lip•ase
- p. C

phos•pho•lip•id

Phos•pho•tec

pho•to•abla•tion
- laser p.

pho•to•che•mo•ther•a•py

pho•to•co•ag•u•la•tion

pho•to•gas•tro•scope

pho•tog•ra•phy
- endoscopic p.
- endoscopic television p.

pho•to•sen•si•ti•za•tion

pho•to•sen•si•tize

pho•to•sen•si•tiz•er

Phys•ick
- P's pouches

phys•i•ol•o•gy
- bolus p.

phys•i•ol•o•gy *(continued)*
  eating p.

phy•to•be•zoar

phy•to•tri•cho•be•zoar

PI
  phosphatidylinositol

pig•ment
  bile p.
  ceroid p.
  early-labeled bile p.
  hepatogenous p.
  late-labeled bile p.
  stool p.

pile
  sentinel p.

piles

pill
  radio p.

pi•lo•be•zoar

pi•lo•car•pine

pin•a•ver•i•um bro•mide

pin•worm

pi•per•a•cil•lin

pi•per•a•zine•di•one

Pip•ra•cil

pir•ox•i•cam

pit
  gastric p's
  p. of the stomach

Pi•tres•sin

PJ
  Peutz-Jeghers syndrome

PJS
  Peutz-Jeghers syndrome

PKC
  protein kinase C

PL
  phospholipid

pir•en•ze•pine

plane
  lateral p., left
  lateral p., right
  subcostal p.
  supracristal p.
  transpyloric p.
  transtubercular p.
  umbilical p.

pla•num *pl.* pla•na
  p. subcostale
  p. transpyloricum

plate
  abdominal flat p.
  ductal p.

Pla•ti•nol

PLC
  phospholipase C

ple•ro•cer•coid

pleu•ro•hep•a•ti•tis

plex•us *pl.* plex•us, plex•us•es
  anterior gastric p.
  Auerbach's p.
  biliary p.
  celiac p.
  p. coeliacus
  colic p., left
  colic p., middle
  colic p., right
  cystic p.
  enteric p.
  p. entericus
  epigastric p.
  esophageal p.
  gastric p's
  p. gastrici
  p. gastricus anterior
  p. gastricus inferior
  p. gastricus posterior
  p. gastricus superior
  gastroepiploic p., left

plex·us *(continued)*
p. haemorrhoidalis
p. haemorrhoidalis medius
p. haemorrhoidalis superior
hemorrhoidal p.
hemorrhoidal p., middle
hemorrhoidal p., superior
hepatic p.
p. hepaticus
ileocolic p.
inferior gastric p.
intermesenteric p.
p. intermesentericus
intestinal p., submucous
intramural p.
lienal p.
p. lienalis
mesenteric p., inferior
mesenteric p., superior
p. mesentericus inferior
p. mesentericus superior
myenteric p.
p. myentericus
p. oesophageus
pancreatic p.
p. pancreaticus
peribiliary vascular p.
periesophageal venous p.
posterior gastric p.
rectal p's, inferior
rectal p's, middle
rectal p., superior
p. rectales inferiores
p. rectales medii
p. rectalis superior
splenic p.
p. splenicus
Stach's p.
submucosal p.
p. submucosus
submucous p.
subserosal p.
p. subserosus
superior gastric p.
p. venosus rectalis
venous p., rectal

pli·ca *pl.* pli·cae
plicae caecales
p. caecalis vascularis
plicae cecales
p. cecalis vascularis
plicae circulares
plicae circulares [Kerkringi]
plicae conniventes
p. duodenalis inferior
p. duodenalis superior
p. duodenojejunalis
p. duodenomesocolica
p. epigastrica peritonaei
plicae gastricae
p. gastropancreatica
p. hepatopancreatica
p. ileocaecalis
p. ileocecalis
p. longitudinalis duodeni
p. paraduodenalis
p. recti
plicae semilunares coli
p. sigmoidea coli
p. spiralis
plicae transversales recti
plicae tunicae mucosae vesicae biliaris
plicae tunicae mucosae vesicae felleae
p. umbilicalis lateralis
plicae villosae gastris
plicae villosae ventriculi

pli·ca·tion
posterior p.
puborectalis p.

plug
bile p.
Gelfoam p.
Vaseline gauze p.

Plum·mer
P.-Vinson syndrome

PMN
polymorphonuclear leukocytes

PMS Ami•trip•ty•line

PMS Me•tro•ni•da•zole

PMS Pro•meth•a•zine

PMS Sul•fa•sal•a•zine

pneu•ma•to•sis
- p. cystoides intestinalis
- p. cystoides intestinorum
- intestinal p.
- p. intestinalis

pneu•mo•bil•ia

pneu•mo•cho•le•cys•ti•tis

pneu•mo•co•lon

pneu•mo•peri•to•ne•um

pneu•mo•peri•to•ni•tis

PNTML
- pudendal nerve terminal motor latency

point
- Boas' p.
- Chauffard's p.
- dorsal p.
- Griffith's p.
- Lanz's p.
- McBurney's p.
- Mackenzie's p.
- Pauly's p.
- phrenic-pressure p.
- Ramond's p.
- Robson's p.

Po•lar en•ter•al feed•ing bag

pol•i•do•can•ol

pol•ox•a•lene

pol•ox•a•mer
- p. 188

Pol•ya
- P. anastomosis
- P. anterior technique
- P's operation
- P. posterior technique

poly•amine

poly•car•bo•phil
- calcium p.

poly•chlo•rin•at•ed bi•phen•yl (PCB)

poly•cho•lia

poly•chy•lia

Poly•cil•lin

Poly•cose cal•o•rie sup•ple•ment

Poly•cose car•bo•hy•drate mod•ule

Poly•dek su•ture

poly•dex•trose

poly•eth•y•lene
- p. glycol

poly•glac•tin
- p. 910

poly I:C

poly•lac•tos•amino•gly•can

Poly•mox

poly•myo•si•tis

pol•yp
- adenomatous p.
- carpet p.
- clamshell p.
- colonic p.
- colorectal p.
- Cronkhite-Canada p.
- diminutive p.
- duodenal p.
- epithelial p.
- extended p.
- fundic gland p.
- gastric p.
- gastrointestinal p.
- giant inflammatory p.
- hamartomatous p.
- hyperplastic p.
- index p.

pol•yp *(continued)*
inflammatory p.
inflammatory fibroid p.
intestinal p.
jejunal p.
juvenile p's
lymphoid p's
malignant p.
marble-type p.
mountain-type p.
multilobulated
pedunculated p.
neoplastic p.
pedunculated p.
periampullary p.
Peutz-Jeghers p.
rectal p.
residual p.
ridge-type p.
sessile p.
squamous p.

poly•pec•to•my
colonoscopic p.
endoscopic p.
piecemeal p.
snare p.

poly•pep•tide
gastric inhibitory p. (GIP)
human pancreatic p.
islet amyloid p.
pancreatic p.
spasmolytic p.
vasoactive intestinal p.
(VIP)

poly•po•sis
acquired multiple p.
adenomatous p.
adenomatous p. coli
p. coli
familial p.
familial adenomatous p.
familial p. coli
familial intestinal p.
filiform p.
gastric p.
p. gastrica

poly•po•sis *(continued)*
hamartomatous p.
intestinal p.
p. intestinalis
juvenile p.
multiple colonic p.
multiple familial p.
p. ventriculi

poly•sac•cha•ride

pons *pl.* pon•tes
p. hepatis

Pon•sky
P.-Gauderer technique

pon•toon

pool
bile acid p.

Poole
P. suction tip
P. suction tube

Pop•pel
P's sign

Pop•per
P.-Schaffner staging (for
primary biliary cirrhosis)

pore
biliary p.

por•phy•ria
chronic hepatic p.
hepatic p.

por•phy•rin

por•phy•ro•bi•lin•o•gen de•
ami•nase

por•ta *pl.* por•tae
p. hepatis
p. omenti
p. of omentum

Por•ta•gen for•mu•la

por•tal
hepatic p.

Por•ta•lac

Por•ter
P. duodenal forceps

por•to•cho•le•cys•tos•tomy
hepatic p.

por•to•en•ter•os•to•my
hepatic p.

po•si•tion
Buie p.
dorsolithotomy p.
Elliot's p.
greater curve p.
jackknife p.
kneeling-squatting p.
Kraske p.
left lateral p.
lithotomy p.
modified Sims p.
prone p.
prone jackknife p.
right anterior p.
right posterior p.
Robson's p.
Sims' p.
supine p.
Trendelenburg's p.

post•gas•trec•to•my

post•mes•en•ter•ic

post•si•nu•soi•dal

pos•ture
Drosin's p's

po•tas•si•um
p. bitartrate and sodium bicarbonate

po•ten•tial
evoked p.
membrane p.
motor unit p.
pacesetter p.

Potts
P. anastomosis forceps
P.-Smith forceps
P.-Smith mouse-tooth tissue forceps

Potts *(continued)*
P.-Smith plain tissue forceps

pouch
Coloplast p.
colostomy p.
disposable p.
drainable p.
FirstChoice Drainable P.
gastric
H-p.
Hartmann's p.
hepatorenal p.
H-shaped p.
ileoanal p.
ileocecal p.
J-p.
J-shaped p.
one-piece p.
ostomy p.
pelvic p.
Physick's p's
postoperative p.
S-p.
S-shaped p.
Sur-Fit p.
two-piece p.
W-p.
Willis' p.
W-shaped p.
Zenker's p.

pouch•itis
refractory p.
segment p.
short-strip p.

pow•der
karaya gum p.

Pow•er
Robinson-Kepler-P. water test

PP
pancreatic polypeptide
postprandial

PPC
paradoxical puborectalis contraction

PPJ
pure pancreatic juice

PPN
partial parenteral nutrition

PR
puborectalis

Pra•der
P.-Willi syndrome

Pratt
P. anoscope
P. crypt hook
P. rectal hook
P. rectal speculum

Pre-At•tain tube feed•ing for•mu•la

pre•cip•i•ta•tion
bile p.

Pre•ci•sion HN pro•tein and cal•o•rie sup•ple•ment

Pre•ci•sion Iso•ton•ic tube feed•ing for•mu•la

Pre•ci•sion LR pro•tein and cal•o•rie sup•ple•ment

Pre•ci•sion LR tube feed•ing for•mu•la

PRED
prednisone

Pred
prednisone

pre•di•ver•tic•u•lar

pred•ni•mus•tine

pred•nis•o•lone

pred•ni•sone

Pre•ges•ti•mil for•mu•la

Pre•lone

Pre•ma•ture En•fa•mil for•mu•la

pre•med•i•ca•tion

prep
bowel p.

prep•a•ra•tion
bowel p.

pre•py•lor•ic

pres•by•esoph•a•gus

pre•ser•va•tion
sphincter p.

pre•si•nu•soi•dal

pres•sure
anal resting p.
anal squeeze p.
crypt p.
portal venous p.
sinusoidal p.
transhepatic parenchymal p.
wedged hepatic vein p.

Pres•syn

pre•ven•tric•u•lus

Pril•o•sec

Pri•max•in

Prin•ci•pen

Pro-50

pro•an•the•line bro•mide

Pro-Ban•thine

probe
Bakes p.
Barr fistula p.
BICAP p.
Buie fistula p.
contact p. tip
Desjardins gall duct p.
Earle rectal p.
Fenger gallstone p.

probe *(continued)*
fistula p.
Fogarty biliary p.
gallstone p.
heater p.
Larry rectal p.
malleable p.
Mayo common duct p.
Medi-Tech bipolar p.
Mixter common duct dilating p.
Ochsner spiral gallstone p.
Olympus CD-3L monopolar p.
palpating p.
pH p.
silver p.
tactile p.
tumor p.
Wasko common duct p.

PROC
procarbazine

Proc
procarbazine

Pro-Cal-Sof

pro•car•ba•zine

pro•ce•dure
Ball p.
Bloodgood p.
blow-hole p.
DuVal p.
emergent Hartmann's p.
Frykman-Goldberg p.
gracilis sling p.
Hartmann's p.
Puestow-Gillesby p.
pull-through p.
Ripstein p.
Turnbull blow-hole p.
Wells p.
Whipple p.

pro•cer•coid

pro•cess
caudate p.

pro•cess *(continued)*
uncinate p. of pancreas
vermiform p.

pro•ces•sus *pl.* pro•ces•sus
p. caudatus hepatis
p. papillaris hepatis
p. uncinatus pancreatis
p. vermiformis

proc•tal•gia
p. fugax

proc•tec•ta•sia

proc•tec•to•my

proc•ten•clei•sis

Proc•ter
P.-Livingstone endoprosthesis

proc•teu•ryn•ter

proc•teu•ry•sis

proc•ti•tis
allergic p.
factitial p.
herpes simplex II p.
radiation p.
ulcerative p.

proc•to•cly•sis

proc•to•coc•cy•pexy

proc•to•co•lec•to•my
total p.

proc•to•co•li•tis
radiation p.

proc•to•co•lon•os•co•py

Proc•to•cort

Proc•to•Cream-HC

proc•to•dyn•ia

proc•to•gen•ic

proc•to•gram
dynamic p.

proc•tog•ra•phy
balloon p.

proc•to•log•ic

proc•tol•o•gist

proc•tol•o•gy

proc•to•pa•ral•y•sis

proc•to•peri•neo•plas•ty

proc•to•peri•ne•or•rha•phy

proc•to•pexy

proc•to•plas•ty

proc•to•ple•gia

proc•to•poly•pus

proc•top•to•sis

proc•tor•rha•gia

proc•tor•rha•phy

proc•tor•rhea

proc•to•scope
Boehm p.
Gabriel p.
Goldbacher p.
Hirschman p.
Hirschman-Martin p.
Kelly p.
Lieberman p.
Montague p.
Newman p.
Pruitt p.
Strauss p.
Turell p.
Tuttle's p.
Vernon-David p.
Welch Allyn p.
Welch Allyn fiberoptic p.
Yeomans p.

proc•tos•co•py

proc•to•sig•moid

proc•to•sig•moi•dec•to•my
transanal abdominal transanal p.

proc•to•sig•moi•di•tis

proc•to•sig•moi•do•scope
rigid p.

proc•to•sig•moi•dos•co•py
flexible p.

proc•to•spasm

proc•tos•ta•sis

proc•to•ste•no•sis

proc•tos•to•my

proc•to•tome

proc•tot•o•my
external p.
internal p.

Pro•di•em

pro•duc•tion
bile p.

pro•en•zyme

Pro•Fi•ber tube feed•ing for•mu•la

pro•file
longitudinal pressure p.

pro•glot•tid

pro•jec•tion
anteroposterior supine p.
Chassard-Lapiné p.
lateral p.
lateral decubitus p.
left lateral erect p.
left posterior oblique p.
posteroanterior p.
prone anteroposterior p.
prone right anterior oblique p.
prone right posteroanterior p.
recumbent posterolateral p.
right anterior oblique p.
right lateral p.
right posterior oblique p.

pro•lapse
- anal p.
- p. of anus
- gastric p.
- rectal p.
- p. of rectum
- p. of stoma
- valve p.

pro•lap•sus
- p. ani
- p. recti

Pro-Lax

Pro•lo•prim

Pro•Max pro•tein mod•ule

Pro•meth

pro•meth•a•zine

Pro•meth•e•gan

Pro-Mix pro•tein mod•ule

Pro-Mix pro•tein sup•ple•ment

Pro•Mod pro•tein mod•ule

Prompt

Pro•pac pro•tein mod•ule

Pro•pan•thel

pro•pan•the•line

pro•pyl•thio•ura•cil

Pro•rex

Pros•kau•er
- Voges-P. test

Pro•So•bee for•mu•la

Pro-Sof

pros•ta•cy•clin

Pros•taph•lin

pros•the•sis *pl.* pros•the•ses
- antireflux p.
- endoscopic p.
- Marlex p.

Pro•stig•min

pro•stig•mine

Pro•ta•min tube feed•ing for•mu•la

pro•tein
- biliary p.
- C p.
- p. C
- calcium-binding p.
- carcinofetal p's
- copper-binding p.
- dietary p.
- fatty acid–binding p.
- G p.
- GP-2 (pancreatic granule) p.
- heat shock p. (Hsp)
- hepatic bile acid transporter p.
- insulin-like growth factor binding p.
- membrane fatty-acid binding p.
- pancreatitis-associated p. (PAP)
- R p.
- retinol-binding p. (RBP)
- p. thiol

pro•tein ki•nase

pro•te•ol•y•sis

Pro•tha•zine

Pro•ti•lase

pro•to•col
- balloon reflex p.
- motility p.

pro•to•du•o•de•num

pro•to•por•phy•rin•o•gen ox•i•dase

Pro•to•stat

Pro•trin

pro•tru•sion
 anal p.

pro•tu•ber•ance
 pigmented p.

Pro•tyl•ol

pro•vi•ta•min

Pru•itt
 P. anoscope
 P. proctoscope

PS
 pyloric stenosis

PSC
 primary sclerosing cholangitis

pseu•do•ap•pen•di•ci•tis
 p. zooparasitica

pseu•do•car•ci•nom•a•tous

pseu•do•cyst
 pancreatic p.

pseu•do•dys•en•tery

pseu•do•hau•stra•tion

pseu•do•in•con•ti•nence

pseu•do•li•thi•a•sis

pseu•do•mega•co•lon

pseu•do•mel•a•no•sis

pseu•do•mem•brane

pseu•do•mem•bra•nous

pseu•do•my•ia•sis

pseu•do-ob•struc•tion
 idiopathic intestinal p.
 intestinal p.

pseu•do•pol•yp
 fundal fold p.

pseu•do•pol•y•po•sis

pseu•do•pty•al•ism

pseu•do•vom•it•ing

psor•en•ter•itis

PSPD
 posterior superior pancreaticoduodenal artery

PSU
 primary site undetermined

psyl•li•um
 p. hydrophilic mucilloid
 malt soup extract and p.
 p. and senna

pter•o•yl•glu•tam•ic acid

PTHBD
 percutaneous transhepatic biliary drainage

PTHC
 percutaneous transhepatic cholangiography

PU
 peptic ulcer

pu•bo•rec•ta•lis

PUD
 peptic ulcer disease

Pues•tow
 Eder-P. dilator
 P.-Gillesby procedure

PUFA
 polyunsaturated fatty acid

Pul•mo•care tube feed•ing for•mu•la

pulse
 hepatic p.

pump
 Biosearch 7000 enteral feeding p.
 Biosearch 7005 enteral feeding p.
 Compat 199205 enteral feeding p.
 Cub R-200 enteral feeding p.

pump *(continued)*
- Dobhoff 8000 enteral feeding p.
- ENtech enteral feeding p.
- enteral p.
- Flexiflo Companion enteral feeding p.
- Flexiflo enteral feeding p.
- Flexiflo II enteral feeding p.
- Flexiflo III enteral feeding p.
- Flogard 2000 enteral feeding p.
- Holter Pediatric P. 903
- Holter Pediatric P. 907
- IMED 430 enteral feeding p.
- infusion p.
- Kangaroo 200 enteral feeding p.
- Kangaroo 324 enteral feeding p.
- Kangaroo 330 enteral feeding p.
- Keofeed 3000 enteral feeding p.
- Keofeed 500 enteral feeding p.
- Keofeed II enteral feeding p.
- KMI 50 enteral feeding p.
- KMI 60 enteral feeding p.
- Nutripro EFS enteral feeding p.
- Simplicity 2100A infusion p.
- stomach p.
- suction p.
- VTR-300 enteral feeding p.

punch
- Murphy p.

pur•ga•tion

purge

pu•rine

pu•rine-nu•cleo•side phos•phor•y•lase

Pu•rine•thol

pu•ro•hep•a•ti•tis

pur•pu•ra
- allergic p.
- anaphylactoid p.
- Henoch's p.
- Henoch-Schönlein p.
- p. nervosa

pus *pl.* pu•ra
- anchovy sauce p.

pu•tres•cine

PV
- portal vein

P&V
- pyloroplasty and vagotomy

PVM Pow•der pro•tein sup•ple•ment

PVM sup•ple•ment

py•em•e•sis

py•lo•ral•gia

py•lo•rec•to•my

py•lo•ric

py•lo•ri•ste•no•sis

py•lo•ro•du•o•de•ni•tis

py•lo•ro•gas•trec•to•my

py•lo•ro•my•ot•o•my
- Fredet-Ramstedt p.

py•lo•ro•plas•ty
- double p.
- Finney p.
- Heineke-Mikulicz p.
- Ramstedt p.

py•lo•ros•co•py

py•lo•ro•spasm
- reflex p.

py•lo•ro•ste•no•sis

py•lo•ros•to•my

py•lo•rot•o•my

py•lo•rus

pyo•che•zia

pyo•fe•cia

Pyo•pen

pyo•peri•to•ne•um

pyo•peri•to•ni•tis

pyo•pneu•mo•cho•le•cys•ti•
tis

pyo•pneu•mo•hep•a•ti•tis

pyo•pneu•mo•peri•to•ne•um

pyo•pneu•mo•peri•to•ni•tis

pyr•i•dox•ine

Py•ro•lite

py•ro•sis

py•ru•vate

py•ru•vate car•box•y•lase

PYY
peptide YY

Q

quad•rant
  left lower q. (LLQ)
  left upper q. (LUQ)
  right lower q. (RLQ)
  right upper q. (RUQ)

Ques•tran

Qui•a•gel PG

Quick
  Q's test

Qui•ess

Quin•ton
  Rubin-Q. small bowel biopsy tube

quo•tient
  respiratory q.

rad•i•cal
free r.

rad•i•cle
hemorrhoidal r.

ra•di•og•ra•phy
air-contrast r.
double contrast r.
spot-film compression r.

ra•dio•ther•a•py
adjuvant r.
contact r.
endocavitary r.
intraoperative r. (IORT)
postoperative r.
preoperative r.

ra•dix *pl.* ra•di•ces
r. mesenterii

RAIR
retroanal inhibitory reflexes

Ra•mond
R's point

Ramp•ley
R. sponge-holding forceps

Ram•stedt
Fredet-R. operation
Fredet-R. pyloromyotomy
R's operation
R. pyloric stenosis dilator
R. pyloroplasty technique

ra•mus *pl.* ra•mi
r. anterior ductus hepatici dextri
r. lateralis ductus hepatici sinistri
r. medialis ductus hepatici sinistri
r. posterior ductus hepatici dextri

Ran•dall
R. stone forceps

ra•ni•ti•dine
r. bismuth citrate

Ran•kin
R. anastomosis clamp
R. clamp
R. intestinal clamp

Ran•son
R. criteria (scale) (for severity of pancreatitis)

ran•u•la
pancreatic r.

ra•pa•my•cin

Rap•a•port
R. common duct dilator

Rap•o•lyte

Rap•pa•port
R. classification (for non-Hodgkin's lymphoma)

ras•pa•to•ry
Doyen r.

rate
basal metabolic r.
basal metabolism r. (BMR)
five-year survival r.
rebleeding r.

ra•tio
cholic acid:chenodeoxy-cholic acid r.
urea-creatinine r.

Rat•liff
R.-Blake gallstone forceps
R.-Mayo gallstone forceps

Raw•son
Abbott-R. tube

ra•zox•ane

RCF for•mu•la

RCS
  red color signs

RDA
  recommended daily allowance
  recommended dietary allowance

RE
  regional enteritis

Re•ab•i•lan HN tube feed•ing for•mu•la

Re•ab•i•lan tube feed•ing for•mu•la

re•a•gent
  Fouchet's r.
  Toepfer's r.

re•bleed•ing

re•cep•tor
  adrenergic r's
  asialoglycoprotein r.
  muscarinic r's
  vasopressinergic r.

re•cess
  gastric r.
  r. of lesser omental cavity
  paracolic r's
  r. of pelvic mesocolon
  phrenicohepatic r's
  subhepatic r's
  subphrenic r's

re•ces•sus *pl.* re•ces•sus
  r. duodenalis inferior
  r. duodenalis superior
  r. duodenojejunalis
  r. hepatorenalis
  r. ileocaecalis inferior
  r. ileocaecalis superior
  r. ileocecalis inferior
  r. ileocecalis superior
  r. inferior omentalis
  r. intersigmoideus
  r. lienalis

re•ces•sus *(continued)*
  r. paracolici
  r. paraduodenalis
  r. phrenicohepatici
  r. retrocaecalis
  r. retrocecalis
  r. retroduodenalis
  r. splenicus
  r. subhepatici
  r. subphrenici
  r. superior omentalis

Re•clo•mide

Re•com•bi•nant HB

Re•com•bi•vax HB

rec•tal

rec•tal•gia

rec•tec•to•my

rec•ti•tis

rec•to•ab•dom•i•nal

rec•to•cly•sis

rec•to•coc•cy•pexy

rec•to•co•li•tis

Rec•to•cort

rec•to•pexy
  mesh r.
  suture r.

rec•to•plas•ty

rec•to•ro•mano•scope

rec•to•ro•ma•nos•co•py

rec•tor•rha•phy

rec•to•scope

rec•tos•co•py

rec•to•sig•moid

rec•to•sig•moi•dec•to•my
  perineal r.

rec•to•ste•no•sis

rec•tos•to•my

rec•to•tome

rec•tot•o•my

rec•tum
defunctionalized r.
prolapse r.

re•cur•rence
local r.

red
Congo r.

red•ness
diffuse r.

REE
resting energy expenditure

re•flec•tion
lateral peritoneal r.
peritoneal r.

re•flex
defecation r.
enterogastric r.
enteropancreatic r.
esophagosalivary r.
faucial r.
gastrocolic r.
gastroileal r.
gastrointestinal (GI) r.
gastropancreatic r.
ileogastric r.
intestinointestinal r.
myenteric r.
peritoneointestinal r.
rectal r.
renointestinal r.
r. retroanal inhibitory
Roger's r.
vesicointestinal r.
visceromotor r.
von Mering r.

re•flux
alkaline r.
bile r.
cholangiovenous r.
duodenogastric r.
gastroesophageal r.

re•gen•er•a•tion
hepatic r.
liver r.

re•gio *pl.* re•gi•o•nes
r. abdominalis
regiones abdominales
r. epigastrica
r. hypochondriaca
r. hypogastrica
r. inguinalis
r. lumbalis
r. lumbaris
r. pubica
r. umbilicalis

re•gion
abdominal r.
epigastric r.
hypochondriac r.
hypogastric r.
inguinal r.
lumbar r.
umbilical r.

Reg•lan

Reg•u•lace

reg•u•la•tion

Reg•u•lax SS

Reg•u•lex

Reg•u•lex-D

Reg•u•loid

Reg•u•tol

Reh•fuss
R. duodenal tube
R. method
R. test
R. tube

Re•hy•dra•lyte

Rei•chert FPS-3 fi•ber•op•tic sig•moido•scope

Rei•chert SC-35 fi•ber•op•tic sig•moido•scope

Rei•chert SC-4B fi•ber•op•tic sig•moido•scope

Rei•chert SC-5 fi•ber•op•tic sig•moido•scope

Reich•mann
R's syndrome

re•jec•tion
transplant r.

re•lapse
ulcer r.

Re•lax•a•don

re•lax•a•tion
muscle r.

Ren•du
Osler-Walker-R. syndrome

Rennes var•i•ant ga•lac•tos•emia

Re•no•graf•in

Re•no•graf•in-30

ren•za•pride

re•pair
Alliston r.
Henry femoral hernia r.
LaRoque r.
Lotheissen femoral hernia r.
McVay r.
transabdominal r.
Usher-Bellis hernia r.

Re•plete tube feed•ing for•mu•la

Rep-Pred

re•sec•tion
abdominoperineal r.
bowel r.
curative r.
endoscopic tumor r.
gastric r.
ileal r.
intestinal r.

re•sec•tion *(continued)*
palliative r.
sigmoid r.
sleeve r.

re•ser•voir
fluid r.
Hays-de Alameida gastric r.
Hoffmann-Steinberg gastric r.
Hunicutt-Lee gastric r.
Hunt–Limo-Basto gastric r.
Lawrence gastric r.
Longmire and Beal gastric r.
State-Moroney gastric r.

res•i•due
amino acid residue
gastric r.

re•sid•u•um *pl.* re•sid•ua
gastric r.

re•sis•tance
multidrug r.

Re•sol

Re•source tube feed•ing for•mu•la

rest
total bowel r.

REST syn•drome

retch•ing

ret•i•noid

ret•i•nol

Re•tor•tam•o•nas

re•trac•tion
r. of stoma

re•trac•tor
Babcock gallbladder r.
Balfour r.
Balfour self-retaining r.
bowel r.

re•trac•tor *(continued)*
Buie-Smith anal r.
Cardillo r.
cat's-paw r.
Cole duodenal r.
Crile r.
Crile malleable r.
Cushing vein r.
Deaver r.
DeBakey-Cooley r.
Ferguson anal r.
Ferguson-Moon rectal r.
Foss gallbladder r.
Franklin flexible r.
Fritsch's r.
gallbladder r.
Gelpi r.
Gosset self-retaining appendectomy r.
Goulet r.
Grant gallbladder r.
half-moon r.
Harrington r.
Harrington splanchnic r.
Helfrick anal r.
Hill-Ferguson r.
Hill-Ferguson rectal r.
Israel r.
Kelly r.
Klemme self-retaining appendectomy r.
Kocher r.
Langenbeck r.
Mayo-Adams self-retaining appendectomy r.
McBurney r.
McBurney appendectomy r.
Miller double-end r.
Morris r.
Murphy r.
Nuttall liver r.
O'Connor r.
O'Connor-O'Sullivan r.
Panting self-retaining abdominal r.
Parker r.

re•trac•tor *(continued)*
Parker ribbon r.
Parker-Mott r.
Percy-Wolfson r.
rake r.
ribbon r.
Richardson r.
Richardson appendectomy r.
Richardson right angle r.
Rigby rectal r.
Rigby self-retaining appendectomy r.
Roux r.
Sawyer rectal r.
self-retaining r.
Senn r.
Smith anal r.
Smith-Buie anal r.
sweetheart r.
Theis self-retaining r.
U.S. r.
vein r.
Volkmann r.
Volkmann rake r.
Walker gallbladder r.
Weinberg r.
Weitlaner r.
Winsbury-White deep r.
Wolfson gallbladder r.
Worrall deep r.

re•triev•er
polyp r.

ret•ro•flex•ion

ret•ro•peri•stal•sis

ret•ro•peri•to•ne•al

ret•ro•ver•sion

ret•ro•vi•rus

Ret•zi•us
R. veins

re•ver•sal
r. of gradient

rhab•do•myo•sar•co•ma

Rhe•a•ban

RHL
right hepatic lobe

RI
regional ileitis

ri•ba•vi•rin

ri•bo•fla•vin

Ri•chard•son
R. appendectomy retractor
R. retractor
R. right angle retractor

Rich•mond
R. thumb tissue forceps

Rich•ner
R.-Hanhart syndrome

Rich•ter
R's hernia

ri•do•grel

Rie•del
R's lobe

Rieux
R's hernia

rif•am•pin

rif•ax•i•mine

Rig•by
R. rectal retractor
R. self-retaining appendectomy retractor

RIH
right inguinal hernia

Ring
R. catheter

ring
A r.
anorectal r.
B r.
crural r.
esophageal r.
femoral r.

ring *(continued)*
multiple esophageal r.
Ochsner's r.
pigmented corneal r.
Schatzki's r.

Ring•er
R's lactate solution

Ri•o•pan

Ri•o•pan Plus

Ri•o•pan Plus 2

rip•ple
peristaltic r.

Rip•stein
R. procedure

RLQ
right lower quadrant

RMC
rectal motor complex

RMS (Ruvalcaba-Myrhe-Smith) syn•drome

RMS Uni•serts

Ro•ba•late

Rob•bers
R. forceps

Rob•i•my•cin

Rob•in•son
R. catheter
R.-Kepler-Power water test

Ro•bi•nul

Rob•son
Mayo-R. gallstone scoop
R's point
R's position

Ro•ceph•in

Ro•ches•ter
R. gallstone forceps
R.-Ochsner forceps
R.-Péan forceps

Roc•key
R.-Davis incision
R.-Davis modification of McBurney incision

rod
colostomy r.
T-r.
Y glass r.

Rof•er•on-A

Ro•ger
R's reflex
R's syndrome

Ro•gers
R. needle holder

Ro•ki•tan•sky
Cushing-R. ulcer
R's diverticulum
R's hernia
R.-Aschoff ducts
R.-Aschoff sinuses
R.-Cushing ulcer

Ro•laids

roll
iliac r.
Kraske r.

ro•mano•scope

Rom•berg
Howship-R. sign

Ro-My•cin

Ron•do•my•cin

Roose•velt
R. gastroenterostomy clamp

rose
r. bengal

Ro•sen•bach
R's sign
R.-Gmelin test

Ro•sen•thal
R's test

ro•sette
hepatocyte r.

Ross•bach
R's disease

Ros•ser
R. crypt hook

Ros•si
R. contraction

ro•ta•vi•rus

Ro•to•lith litho•trite

Ro•tor
R. syndrome

Rou•bac

round•worm

Roux
R. loop
R. retractor
R.-en-Y anastomosis
R.-en-Y jejunostomy
R.-en-Y operation

Ro•vi•ghi
R's sign

Rov•sing
R's sign

Ro•wa•sa

Rox•a•nol

RP
resting pressure

RQ
respiratory quotient

RR
renin release

RRR
renin-release rate

Ru•bex

ru•bid•a•zone

Ru•bin
R.-Quinton small bowel biopsy tube

ruc•tus

ru•ga *pl.* ru•gae
rugae gastricae
rugae of stomach

Rug•by
R. deep surgery forceps

ru•gi•tus

Ru•lox

Ru•lox No. 1

Ru•lox No. 2

RUOQ
right upper outer quadrant

rup•ture
hepatic r.

RUQ
right upper quadrant

rush
peristaltic r.

Rus•sell
R. technique

Rus•sian for•ceps

Ru•val•ca•ba
R.-Myrhe-Smith syndrome

Ruysch
R's disease

RWM
red wale marking

ry•a•no•dine

Ryle
R. duodenal tube
R's tube

sac
  epiploic s.
  greater s. of peritoneum
  hernial s.
  lesser s. of peritoneal cavity
  omental s.
  splenic s.

sac•cu•la•tion
  s's of colon
  haustral s's

Sacks
  S.-Vine technique

Safe-T-Flex en•ter•al feed•ing con•tain•er

Sah•li
  S's glutoid test
  S's test
  S.-Nencki test

Saint
  S's triad

St. Jo•seph An•ti•di•ar•rhe•al

Sal•a•zo•py•rin

sal•bu•ta•mol

sal•i•cyl•a•zo•sul•fa•pyr•i•dine

sa•line
  hypertonic s.

sa•li•va

Sal•mon
  S. backcut incision

Sal•mo•nel•la
  S. agona
  S. choleraesuis
  S. choleraesuis var. *kuzendorf*

Sal•mo•nel•la (continued)
  S. choleraesuis var. *typhisuis*
  S. enteritidis
  S. enteritidis serotype *agona*
  S. enteritidis serotype *heidelberg*
  S. enteritidis serotype *hirschfeldii*
  S. enteritidis serotype *infantis*
  S. enteritidis serotype *newport*
  S. enteritidis serotype *schottmuelleri*
  S. heidelberg
  S. hirschfeldii
  S. infantis
  S. newport
  S. paratyphi
  S. paratyphi A
  S. paratyphi B
  S. paratyphi C
  S. typhi

sal•mo•nel•la *pl.* sal•mo•nel•lae

Sal•o•falk

salt
  bile s's

sand
  intestinal s.

San•ders
  S. incision

San•di•fer
  S's syndrome

Sani-Supp

San•to•ri•ni
  S's canal
  duct of S.

San•to•ri•ni *(continued)*
major caruncle of S.
papilla of S.

Sap•pey
accessory portal system of S.

sar•coi•do•sis
hepatic s.

sar•co•ma *pl.* sar•co•mas, sar•co•ma•ta
Boeck's s.
Kaposi's s.

Sa•ri•sol No. 2

Sar•ot
S. needle holder

SART
standard acid reflux testing

S.A.S.

S.A.S.-500

S.A.S. En•ter•ic

sa•ti•e•ty
postprandial s.

Sa•tin•sky
S. clamp

sau•cer•ize

Sa•va•ry
S. bougie
S. dilator
S.-Gilliard dilator
S.-Miller scale (for esophagitis)

Sa•wa•gu•chi
S. operation

Saw•yer
S. rectal retractor
S. rectal speculum

SB
serum bilirubin
small bowel

SBFT
small bowel follow through

SBO
small bowel obstruction

scale
French s.
Graham s. (for drug-induced gastric mucosal damage)
Lanza s. (for drug-induced gastric mucosal damage)
modified Lanza s. (for drug-induced gastric mucosal damage)
Ranson s. (for pancreatitis)
Savary-Miller s. (for esophagitis)

scal•lop•ing

scan
gallium-67 s.
liver-spleen s.
milk s.

scan•ning
^{14}Cr-albumin s.
indium-111 leukocyte s.
radionuclide s.

scato•log•ic

sca•tol•o•gy

sca•to•ma

scat•ter•ing
dye s.

SCFA
short-chain fatty acid

Schaff•ner
Popper-S. staging (for primary biliary cirrhosis)

Schat•zki
S's ring

Scheu•er

Scheu•er *(continued)*
S. staging (for primary biliary cirrhosis)

Schiff
S's biliary cycle

Schil•ling
S. test

Schin•dler
S. gastroscope
Wolf-S. gastroscope

Schis•to•so•ma
S. haematobium
S. intercalatum
S. japonicum
S. mansoni

schis•to•so•ma•ci•dal

schis•to•so•ma•cide

schis•to•so•mal

schis•to•some

schis•to•so•mi•a•sis
hepatic s.
s. intercalatum
intestinal s.
s. japonica
Manson's s.
s. mansoni
Oriental s.
visceral s.

schis•to•so•mi•ci•dal

schis•to•so•mi•cide

Schnidt
S. clamp
S. gall duct forceps

Schoe•ma•ker
S. anastomosis
S.-Billroth II technique

Schoen•berg
S. intestinal forceps

Schön•lein
Henoch-S. purpura

Schön•lein *(continued)*
Henoch-S. syndrome
S.-Henoch disease
S.-Henoch purpura
S.-Henoch syndrome

Schultz
triad of S.

schwan•no•ma

Schwartz
Watson-S. test

scin•tig•ra•phy

scin•ti•pho•to•sple•no•por•tog•ra•phy

scis•sors
Bard-Parker s.
Brooks gallbladder s.
Buie rectal operating s.
Busch umbilical s.
Church deep surgery s.
Classon deep surgery s.
Crafoord thoracic s.
Deaver operating s.
Doyen abdominal s.
Duffield deep surgery s.
Ferguson abdominal s.
Fulton deep surgery s.
Graham deep surgery s.
Harrington-Mayo s.
Hooper deep surgery s.
Jorgenson dissecting s.
Lahey s.
Lincoln deep surgery s.
Litwin angled s.
Mayo s.
Mayo straight and curved s.
Mayo-Noble dissecting s.
McIndoe long s.
Metzenbaum s.
Miller rectal operating s.
Nelson s.
Panzer gallbladder s.
plastic straight and curved blunt s.
Sistrunk dissecting s.

scis•sors *(continued)*
- Thorek dissecting s.
- Willauer thoracic s.

scle•ro•der•ma

scle•ro•sant

scle•ro•sis
- gastric s.
- injection s.

scle•ro•ther•a•py
- esophageal variceal s. (EVS)
- injection s.

sco•lex *pl.* sco•le•ces

scoop
- Beck s.
- Desjardins gallstone s.
- Ferguson gallstone s.
- Ferris common duct s.
- gallstone s.
- Klebanoff gallstone s.
- Luer-Korte gallstone s.
- malleable s.
- Mayo common duct s.
- Mayo cystic duct s.
- Mayo gallstone s.
- Mayo-Robson gallstone s.
- Moore gallstone s.
- Moynihan gallstone probe and s.

scope
- Jesberg s.

sco•pol•a•mine
- atropine, hyoscyamine, s., and phenobarbital
- s. butylbromide
- hyoscyamine and s.
- hyoscyamine, s., and phenobarbital

screen
- Marlex s.

screen•ing

scro•to•cele

scyb•a•la

scyb•a•lous

scyb•a•lum *pl.* scyb•a•la

seat•worm

se•cret•a•gogue
- macrophage-derived mucin s.

se•cre•tin

se•cre•tion
- acid s.
- bile s.
- intestinal s.

seg•ment
- hepatic s's
- s's of liver
- vaterian s.

seg•men•ta•tion
- haustral s.

seg•men•tum *pl.* seg•men•ta
- segmenta hepatis

Seid•litz
- S. powder test

se•le•ni•um

Se•les•to•ject

se•mus•tine

Se•nex•on

Seng•sta•ken
- S.-Blakemore tube

Senn
- S. retractor
- Stamm-S. gastroscopy (Billroth type)

sen•na
- s. and docusate
- psyllium and s.
- psyllium hydrophilic mucilloid and s.

sen•no•side

sen•no•sides
psyllium hydrophilic mucilloid and s.

Sen•o•kot

Sen•o•lax

sen•sa•tion
anorectal s.

sen•si•tiv•i•ty
gluten s.

sep•a•ra•tor
Benson pylorus s.

sep•sis

Sep•tra

sep•tum *pl.* sep•ta
fibrous s.

Ser•a•fi•ni
S's hernia

Se•reen

se•ries
small intestinal s.
UGI (upper gastrointestinal) s.

se•ro•co•li•tis

se•ro•en•te•ri•tis

se•ro•mus•cu•lar

se•ro•sa

sero•to•nin

Se•ru•tan

ses•sile

set
Birtcher procto-sigmoid desiccation s.
Boehm rectal diagnostic and treatment s.
Brunner ligature s.
Freiburg biopsy s.
Kangaroo Feeding S.

set *(continued)*
Stone-Holcombe intestinal clamp s.
Welch Allyn rectal s.

se•ton

SFEMG
single fiber electromyography

SFM sta•pler

S-14 for•mu•la

Shall•cross
S. cystic duct forceps

sham-feed•ing

shears
Bethune s.
Lebsche s.

sheath
overtube s.

sheet
Marlex s.

shelf
mesocolic s.

Shi•gel•la
S. ambigua
S. arabinotarda type A
S. arabinotarda type B
S. boydii
S. dysenteriae
S. flexneri
S. newcastle
S. paradysenteriae
S. schmitzii
S. shigae
S. sonnei

Shin•er
S's tube

shunt
cholehepatic s.
Denver s.
LeVeen s.
Linton s.

shunt *(continued)*
- mesocaval s.
- peritoneovenous s.
- portacaval s.
- portal-systemic s.
- side-to-side portacaval s.
- splenorenal s.
- splenorenal s., distal
- Warren s.

shunt•ing
- cholehepatic s.

si•alo•gas•trone

si•alo•mu•cin

si•al•yl•trans•fer•ase

Sib•lin

sid•er•o•sis
- hepatic s.

Sif•fert
- S. method

sig•moid

sig•moid•ec•to•my

sig•moid•itis

sig•moido•pexy

sig•moido•proc•tos•to•my

sig•moido•rec•tos•to•my

sig•moido•scope
- ACMI T915 fiberoptic s.
- ACMI TX915 fiberoptic s.
- Boehm s.
- Buie s.
- fiberoptic s.
- flexible s.
- Fujinon PRO-PC fiberoptic s.
- Fujinon SIG-E2 fiberoptic s.
- Fujinon SIG-PC fiberoptic s.
- Kelly s.
- Lieberman s.
- Montague s.

sig•moido•scope *(continued)*
- Olympus CF-ITS2 fiberoptic s.
- Olympus CPF-P10-S fiberoptic s.
- Olympus OSF-35 fiberoptic s.
- Olympus OSF-60 fiberoptic s.
- Pentax FS-34A fiberoptic s.
- Reichert FPS-3 fiberoptic s.
- Reichert SC-35 fiberoptic s.
- Reichert SC-4B fiberoptic s.
- Reichert SC-5 fiberoptic s.
- rigid s.
- Solow s.
- Strauss s.
- Turell s.
- Tuttle s.
- Vernon-David s.
- Welch Allyn 80055 fiberoptic s.
- Welch Allyn s.
- Yeomans s.

sig•moido•scop•ic

sig•moid•os•co•py
- fiberoptic s.
- flexible s.
- rigid s.

sig•moido•sig•moi•dos•to•my

sig•moid•os•to•my

sig•moid•ot•o•my

sign
- antral pad s.
- bald fundus s.
- Blumberg's s.
- Boyce's s.
- Carman-Kirklin meniscus s.
- colon cut-off s.
- common duct s.

sign *(continued)*
- Cope's s.
- Courvoisier's s.
- crumpled haustrum s.
- Cullen's s.
- double-bubble s.
- double-duct s.
- double-track s.
- s. of the duct
- duodenal cut-off s.
- Federici's s.
- flank stripe s.
- Frostberg's reversed 3 s.
- Gilbert's s.
- Grey Turner's s.
- hairbrush s.
- H bomb s.
- Henning's s.
- Horn's s.
- Howship-Romberg s.
- inverted 3 sign
- Lennhoff's s.
- McBurney's s.
- Meltzer's s.
- Mercedes-Benz s.
- Mexican hat s.
- Murphy's s.
- Naclerio's s.
- obturator s.
- pad s.
- palisade s.
- Pfuhl's s.
- Poppel's s.
- pseudokidney s.
- psoas s.
- psoas and obturator s.
- ram's horn s.
- red color s's
- red ring s.
- Rosenbach's s.
- Rovighi's s.
- Rovsing's s.
- sigmoid elevator s.
- small bowel s.
- smooth greater curvature s.

sign *(continued)*
- sonographic Murphy's s.
- Soresi's s.
- squeeze s.
- Stierlin's s.
- string s.
- string of beads s.
- Trimadeau's s.
- Turner's s.
- twisted taper s.
- V s. of Neclario
- wide-mouth diverticula s.
- wind-sock s.

Si•lain-Gel

Silk Bul•let feed•ing tube

Silk Pill feed•ing tube

Silk Tip feed•ing tube

Sil•ver•man
- Franklin-S. biopsy cannula
- Vim-S. needle
- Vim-S. technique

si•ly•mar•in

SIM 2 cath•e•ter

Sim•aal Gel

Sim•aal 2 Gel

si•meth•i•cone
- s., alumina, calcium carbonate, and magnesia
- alumina, magnesia, and s.
- calcium carbonate and s.
- calcium carbonate, magnesia, and s.
- magaldrate and s.

Sim•i•lac for•mu•la

Sim•i•lac Spe•cial Care for•mu•la

Sim•mons
- S. catheter

Sim•plic•i•ty 2100A in•fu•sion pump

Sims
- S. anoscope
- S. position
- S. rectal speculum

sim•va•sta•tin

Sin•e•quan

Sing•ley
- S. intestinal ring clamp

si•nus *pl.* si•nus, si•nus•es
- anal s's
- s. anales
- s. of Morgagni
- rectal s's
- s. rectales
- Rokitansky-Aschoff s's

si•nu•soi•dal

Sip•py
- S. diet
- S. method
- S. treatment

si•qua

Sis•ter Jo•seph
- S.J.'s nodule

Sis•trunk
- S. dissecting scissors

site
- bleeding s.

si•tos•ter•ol

Sjö•gren
- S's syndrome

Sla•ter
- Bearn-Kunkel-S. syndrome

sleeve
- Williams overtube s.

slip•page
- valve s.

sludge
- biliary s.

SMA
- superior mesenteric artery

SMA for•mu•la

smear
- peripheral blood s.
- potassium hydroxide s.

Smith
- Dixon-Thomas-S. colon clamp
- Potts-S. forceps
- Potts-S. mouse-tooth tissue forceps
- Potts-S. plain tissue forceps
- Ruvalcaba-Myrhe-S. syndrome
- S. anal retractor
- S. electrode
- S. forceps
- S.-Buie anal retractor

SMZ-TMP

snare
- Frankfeldt rectal s.
- long-nose retriever s.
- Norwood rectal s.
- polyp s.
- polypectomy s.
- rectal s.
- wire s.

Sny•der
- S. deep surgery forceps

SO
- sphincter of Oddi

Soave
- S. operation

Soda Mint

so•di•um
- acetaminophen, s. bicarbonate, and citric acid
- alumina, magnesium trisilicate, and s. bicarbonate
- aspirin, s. bicarbonate, and citric acid
- s. bicarbonate

so•di•um *(continued)*
s. chromate Cr 51
magnesium carbonate and s. bicarbonate
s. morrhuate
s. pertechnetate Tc 99m
s. phosphate
potassium bitartrate and s. bicarbonate
s. (pyro- and trimeta-) phosphates
s. tetradecyl sulfate

so•di•um-po•tas•si•um aden•o•sine•tri•phos•pha•tase

Soe•hen•dra
S. Billroth II sphincterotome

soft•en•er
stool s.

soft•en•ing
s. of the stomach

Sol•fo•ton

Sol•i•um

Sol•ow
S. sigmoidoscope

Solu-Cor•tef

Solu-Med•rol

so•lu•tion
balanced electrolyte s.
Carolina rinse s.
Hartman's s.
hypertonic saline s.
lavage s.
Lugol's s.
Ringer's lactate s.
short-chain fatty acid s.

So•ma
S. sphincterotome

so•ma•to•stat•in

Sonne
S. dysentery

so•nog•ra•phy

sor•bin

sor•bi•tol

sor•des
s. gastricae

So•re•sis
S. sign

Soulle
Laubry-S. syndrome

sound
esophageal s.

SP
squeeze pressure
substance P
strictureplasty

sp act
specific activity

space
chyle s's
Disse's s's
extraperitoneal s.
ischiorectal s.
Kiernan's s's
left subphrenic s.
Lesgaft's s.
s. of Mall
perisinusoidal s's
retrorectal s.
right subhepatic s.
right subphrenic s.
sinusoidal s.

spar•ga•no•sis

spar•ga•num *pl.* spar•ga•na

Spas•lin

spasm
diffuse esophageal s.
esophageal s.

Spas•mo•ban

Spas•mo•ject

Spas•mol•in

Spas•mo•phen

Spas•quid

Spas•to•sed

spa•ti•um *pl.* spa•tia
  s. extraperitoneale

Spec•tro•bid

spec•tros•co•py
  fluorescence s.
  magnetic resonance s.

spec•u•lum *pl.* spec•u•la
  Brinkerhoff's s.
  Brinkerhoff rectal s.
  Chelsea-Eaton anal s.
  Cook's s.
  David rectal s.
  Kelly's s.
  Martin's s.
  Martin and Davy s.
  Mathews' s.
  Pratt rectal s.
  Sawyer rectal s.
  Sims' rectal s.
  Vernon-David rectal s.

Spen•cer
  S's disease

Spen•cer Wells
  S.W. forceps

sphinc•ter
  anal s.
  s. ani
  artificial anal s.
  s. of Boyden
  cardiac s.
  cardioesophageal s.
  electrically stimulated gracilis neoanal s.
  external anal s.
  gastroesophageal s.
  Giordano's s.
  s. of hepatopancreatic ampulla
  Hyrtl's s.
  ileocolonic s.
  internal anal s.
  lower esophageal s.
  Lütkens' s.
  Nélaton's s.
  O'Beirne's s.
  s. of Oddi
  Oddi's s.
  pharyngoesophageal s.
  prepyloric s.
  pyloric s.
  rectal s.
  upper esophageal s.

sphinc•ter•is•mus

sphinc•ter•itis

sphinc•tero•plas•ty
  apposition s.
  overlapping s.

sphinc•tero•scope
  Kelly's s.

sphinc•tero•tome
  Billroth II s.
  Doubilet s.
  needle-knife s.
  precut s.
  pull-type s.
  push-type s.
  sigmoid-shaped s.
  Soehendra Billroth II s.
  Soma s.
  traction-type s.

sphinc•ter•ot•o•my
  endoscopic s. (ES)
  internal s.
  lateral internal s.
  multiple anal s's
  partial internal s.
  partial posterior s.

spi•ro•ger•ma•ni•um

splanch•no•lith

splanch•nop•a•thy

splanch•no•tribe

sponge
- gauze s.
- lap s.
- laparotomy s.
- peanut s.
- s. stick

spoon
- Falk appendectomy s.
- gall duct s.
- gallbladder s.
- Moore gallbladder s.

spot
- cherry-red s.
- epigastric s.
- hematocystic s.
- milk s's
- tendinous s's

Sprinz
- Dubin-S. disease
- Dubin-S. syndrome
- S.-Dubin syndrome
- S.-Nelson syndrome

sprue
- celiac s.
- collagenous s.
- non-tropical s.
- refractory s.
- tropical s.
- unclassified s.

spu•tum
- s. aeroginosum
- green s.
- icteric s.

squeeze
- station s.

Ssa•ba•ne•jew
- S.-Frank operation

ST
- stable toxin
- stomach

stag•ing
- AJCC/UICC s. (for colorectal cancer)
- Astler-Coller s. (for colorectal carcinoma)
- Jass s. (for rectal carcinoma)
- Popper-Schaffner s. (for primary biliary cirrhosis)
- Scheuer s. (for primary biliary cirrhosis)
- TNM s.

stain
- Gram's s.
- Papanicolaou's s.
- reticulin s.
- Sudan III s.
- Warthin-Starry silver s.

stain•ing
- in vivo dye s.

stalk
- hemorrhoidal s.

Stamm
- S. gastrostomy
- S.-Senn gastroscopy (Billroth type)

stand
- Mayo s.

Staph•cil•lin

Staph•y•lo•coc•cus
- *S. aureus*

sta•pler
- circular s.
- circular intraluminal s.
- EEA (end-to-end anastomosis) s.
- GIA (gastrointestinal anastomosis) s.
- ligating and dividing s. (LDS)
- linear s.
- linear-cutting s.
- SFM (skin and fascia) s.
- TA (thoracoabdominal) s.

sta•pler *(continued)*
TA-30 s.
TA-55 s.
TA-90 s.

sta•pling
gastric s.

starch

Starck
S. dilator

Star•ry
Warthin-S. stain

star•va•tion

sta•sis
cholate s.
ileal s.
intestinal s.

State
S. operation
S.-Moroney gastric reservoir

state
fasted s.
fed s.
interdigestive s.
postabsorptive s.

Sta•tex

STC
subtotal colectomy

ste•ar•rhea

ste•a•tor•rhea
idiopathic s.

ste•a•to•sis
hepatic s.

Stein•berg
Hoffman-S. gastric reservoir

Ste•met•ic

ste•no•sis
anal s.
bile duct s.

ste•no•sis *(continued)*
hypertrophic pyloric s.
papillary s.
pyloric s.
stomal s.

stent
Amsterdam s.
double pigtail s.
pigtail s.

stent•ing

ster•co•bi•lin

ster•co•bi•lin•o•gen

ster•co•lith

ster•co•ra•ceous

ster•co•ral

ster•co•ro•lith

ster•co•ro•ma

ster•co•rous

ster•cus *pl.* ster•co•ra

stern•zel•len

ste•roid
anabolic s.

Stet•ton
S. spur crusher

Ste•wart
S. crypt hook
S. stitches

stibo•glu•co•nate so•di•um

stick
sponge s.

Stier•lin
S's sign

stitch
Gambee s.
Stewart s's
U s.

Stok•vis
S.-Talma syndrome

sto•ma *pl.* sto•mas, sto•ma•ta
dusky s.
end-loop s.
intestinal s.
loop s.

stom•ach
aberrant umbilical s.
bilocular s.
cardiac s.
dumping s.
fishhook-shaped s.
hourglass s.
leather bottle s.
sclerotic s.
thoracic s.
trifid s.
upside-down s.
waterfall s.
watermelon s.
water-trap s.

stom•a•chal

sto•mach•ic

Sto•ma•he•sive

sto•mal

sto•ma•ta

sto•ma•tal

sto•ma•ti•tis *pl.* sto•ma•tit•i•des
tropical s.

Stone
S. closing forceps
S. intestinal clamp
S.-Holcombe intestinal clamp set

stone
cholesterol s.
pancreatic s.
pigment s.
retained s.

stool
bilious s.
fatty s.

stool *(continued)*
lienteric s.
mucous s.
pipe-stem s.
ribbon s.
sago-grain s.

stool soft•en•er

stop
needle s.

strap
Montgomery s's

Stratte
S. needle holder

stra•tum *pl.* stra•ta
s. circulare gastris
s. circulare tunicae muscularis coli
s. circulare tunicae muscularis intestini tenuis
s. circulare tunicae muscularis recti
s. circulare tunicae muscularis ventriculi
s. circulare ventriculi
s. longitudinale gastris
s. longitudinale tunicae muscularis coli
s. longitudinale tunicae muscularis intestini tenuis
s. longitudinale tunicae muscularis recti
s. longitudinale tunicae muscularis ventriculi
s. longitudinale ventriculi
submucous s. of colon
submucous s. of rectum
submucous s. of small intestine
submucous s. of stomach

Strauss
Payer-S. contraction
S. proctoscope
S. sigmoidoscope

Strep•to•coc•cus

strep•to•my•cin

strep•to•ni•grin

strep•to•zo•cin

stress
  psychologic s.

Stres•stein stress for•mu•la

stric•ture
  benign s.
  biliary s.
  cancerous s.
  esophageal s.
  inflammatory s.
  malignant s.
  neoplastic s.
  postoperative s.
  radiation-induced s.
  stoma s.

stric•ture•plas•ty
  Finney s.
  Heineke-Mikulicz s.
  multiple s's

strip
  Vaseline gauze s.

stripe
  flank s.

strip•ping
  mucosal s.

Stron•gy•loi•des
  S. stercoralis

stron•gy•loi•di•a•sis

stron•gy•loi•do•sis

STS
  sodium tetradecylsulfate

stu•dy
  double-contrast s.
  full-column barium s.
  lactose-barium small bowel s.
  motility s.

stu•dy *(continued)*
  pneumocolon s.
  transit s.

Stu•lex

stump
  rectal s.

sty•let

STZ
  streptozocin

Stz
  streptozocin

sub•en•do•scope

sub•en•do•scop•ic

sub•ic•ter•ic

sub•stance
  s. P

suc•cus *pl.* suc•ci
  s. entericus
  s. gastricus
  s. pancreaticus

su•cral•fate

su•crase

suc•rase iso•mal•tase

su•crose

suc•tion
  Cameron-Miller s.-coagulator
  Harris tube s.
  Wangensteen s.

suc•tion tip
  Andrews s.t.
  Buie rectal s.t.
  Poole s.t.

Su•deck
  S. atrophy

sul•bac•tam
  ampicillin and s.

Sul•crate

sul•cus *pl.* sul•ci
- angular s.
- s. intermedius gastricus
- paracolic sulci
- sulci paracolici
- s. of vena cava
- s. venae cavae

Sul•fa•meth•o•prim

sul•fa•meth•ox•a•zole
- s. and trimethoprim

Sul•fa•prim

sul•fa•sal•a•zine

Sul•fa•trim

sul•fo•bro•mo•phthal•e•in

sul•fo•mu•cin

sul•fon•amide

Sul•fox•a•prim

sul•in•dac

Su•ma•cal car•bo•hy•drate mod•ule

Su•my•cin

Su•per•Char

su•per•ox•ide dis•mu•tase

sup•ple•ment
- Cal Powder calorie s.
- calorie s.
- Case Powder protein s.
- Controlyte calorie s.
- Enrich protein and calorie s.
- Ensure protein and calorie s.
- Flexical Citrotein protein and calorie s.
- Hy-Cal calorie s.
- Isocal protein and calorie s.
- Magnacal protein and calorie s.
- nutritional s.

sup•ple•ment *(continued)*
- Polycose calorie s.
- Precision HN protein and calorie s.
- Precision LR protein and calorie s.
- Pro-Mix protein s.
- PVM Powder protein s.
- Travasorb protein and calorie s.
- vitamin s.
- Vivonex protein and calorie s.

sup•port
- intensive nutritional s.
- nutritional s.

sup•pos•i•to•ry
- hydrocortisone s.

Su•prax

su•ra•min

sur•face
- absorptive s.
- anterior s. of stomach
- diaphragmatic s. of liver
- left diaphragmatic s. of liver
- posterior s. of stomach
- right diaphragmatic s. of liver
- visceral s. of liver

sur•fac•tant

Sur•fak

Sur-Fit pouch

Sur•ga•loy su•ture

sur•gery
- abdominal s.
- anorectal s.
- bariatric s.
- colorectal s.
- intestinal s.
- laser s.

Sur•gi•cel

Sur·gi·lon su·ture

Sur·mon·til

Su·ru·ga
S. operation

Su·sa·no

Sus·ta·cal tube feed·ing for·mu·la

sus·ten·tac·u·lum *pl.* sus·ten·tac·u·la
s. lienis

su·ture
absorbable s.
Albert's s.
Albert-Lembert s.
Appolito's s.
atraumatic catgut s.
atraumatic chromic s.
black silk s.
Bonnell s.
button s.
catgut s.
chromic catgut s.
chromic gut s.
circular s.
Connell s.
continuous s.
cotton s.
Cushing s.
Czerny's s.
Czerny interrupted s.
Czerny-Lembert s.
Dacron s.
Dermalene s.
Dermalon s.
Dexon s.
double-button s.
double-loop mass closure s.
Dupuytren's s.
echelon s.
Ethibond s.
Ethilon s.
everting s.
far-and-near s.
far-near, near-far s.
figure-of-eight s.

su·ture *(continued)*
furrier's s.
Gély's s.
glover's s.
Gould inverted mattress s.
Gussenbauer's s.
Halsted s.
Halsted interrupted mattress s.
Halsted interrupted quilt s.
interrupted s.
inverting s.
Ivalon s.
Lang s.
Lembert s.
Lembert s., continuous
Lembert s., interrupted
lock-stitch s.
Marshall U-stitch s.
Marshall W s.
mattress s., continuous
mattress s., end-on
mattress s., horizontal
mattress s., interrupted
mattress s., inverted
mattress s., on-edge
mattress s., right-angle
Mersilene s.
nylon s.
over-and-over s.
Parker-Kerr s.
Parker-Kerr chromic s.
Perma-Hand s.
plain catgut s.
plain gut s.
Polydek s.
polyester s.
polyethylene s.
pulley s.
pursestring s.
quilt s.
retention s.
running s.
seromuscular s.
silk s.
stainless steel s.
stay s.

su•ture *(continued)*
subcuticular s.
Surgaloy s.
surgical steel s.
Surgilon s.
Tevdek s.
through-and-through s.
through-and-through U-stitch s.
Ti-Cron s.
Tom Jones near-and-far s.
transfixion s.
transition s.
Tycron s.
U-shaped continuous s.
Vicryl s.

swal•low
barium s.

swal•low•ing

Swen•son
S's operation

Syl•lact

Syl•la•malt

symp•tom
obstructive s's

syn•cho•lia

syn•drome (see also under *disease*)
Aagenaes s.
acquired immunodeficiency s. (AIDS)
afferent loop s.
Alagille's s.
bacterial overgrowth s.
Barrett's s.
Bearn-Kunkel s.
Bearn-Kunkel-Slater s.
bile plug s.
blind loop s.
Boerhaave's s.
bowel bypass s.
Budd-Chiari s.
cancer family s.

syn•drome *(continued)*
carcinoid s.
cathartic colon s.
celiac s.
cerebrohepatorenal s.
Charcot's s.
Chiari's s.
Chilaiditi s.
colon coagulation s.
Courvoisier-Terrier s.
Cowden's s.
CREST s.
Crigler-Najjar s.
Cronkhite-Canada s.
Cruveilhier-Baumgarten s.
Dubin-Johnson s.
Dubin-Sprinz s.
dumping s.
Ellis-van Creveld s.
endocrine ulcer s.
familial colon cancer s.
Fitz-Hugh–Curtis s.
flat adenoma s.
Gardner's s.
Gee-Herter-Heubner s.
Gilbert s.
Hanot's s.
Henoch-Schönlein s.
hepatopulmonary s.
hepatorenal s.
hereditary flat adenoma s.
hereditary nonpolyposis colorectal cancer s.
hyperviscosity s.
inspissated bile s.
irritable bowel s.
irritable colon s.
Ivemark's s.
jejunal s.
Jeune's s.
Kunkel's s.
Laubry-Soulle s.
levator s.
levator ani s.
liver-kidney s.
Lynch s. (I and II)
malabsorption s.
Mallory-Weiss s.

syn•drome *(continued)*
- malnutrition s.
- Meckel-Gruber s.
- meconium plug s.
- megacystis-microcolon–intestinal hypoperistalsis s. (MMIHS)
- Menkes' s.
- Mirizzi s.
- multiple hamartoma s.
- nonrelaxing puborectalis s.
- Ogilvie's s.
- Oldfield's s.
- Osler-Rendu-Walker s.
- pancreatic cholera s.
- pancreaticohepatic s.
- pericolic-membrane s.
- Peutz-Jeghers s.
- Plummer-Vinson s.
- polyangiitis overlap s.
- postcholecystectomy s.
- postcolonoscopy distention s.
- postgastrectomy s.
- pouchitis s.
- Prader-Willi s.
- Reichmann's s.
- REST s.
- Richner-Hanhart s.
- Roger's s.
- Rotor's s.
- roux-en-Y s.
- Ruvalcaba-Myhre-Smith s.
- Sandifer's s.
- Schönlein-Henoch s.
- short-bowel s.
- short-gut s.
- Sjögren's s.
- small left colon s.
- solitary rectal ulcer s.
- spastic pelvic floor s.
- splenic flexure s.
- Sprinz-Dubin s.
- Sprinz-Nelson s.
- stagnant loop s.
- stasis s.
- steak house s.

syn•drome *(continued)*
- Stokvis-Talma s.
- sump s.
- superior mesenteric artery s.
- Torkelson s.
- tropical diarrhea-malabsorption s.
- Turcot s.
- Verner-Morrison s.
- wasting s.
- WDHA s.
- Zanca's s.
- Zellweger s.
- Zollinger-Ellison s.

syn•ech•ten•ter•ot•o•my

sy•ringe
- Asepto s.
- Luer-Lok s.

sys•tem
- accessory portal s. of Sappey
- alimentary s.
- BICAP hemostatic s.
- bile collecting s.
- Compat Enteral Delivery S.
- digestive s.
- Ethox/Barron 2000 Feeding Pump S.
- Flexiflo Top-Fill Enteral Nutrition S.
- kallikrein-kinin s.
- Kangaroo Delivery S.
- manovolumetry s.
- Olympus/Aloka GF-EU1/EU-M1 ultrasound endoscopic s.
- portal venous s.
- pouching s.
- VideoEndoscope s.
- Vivonex Acutrol Enteral Feeding S.

sys•te•ma
- s. digestorium

T

TA
 tubular adenoma

ta•ble
 Maquet endoscopy t.

TAC
 total abdominal colectomy

tache
 t. blanche

tachy•gas•tria

TAC/IRA
 total abdominal colectomy with ileorectal anastomosis

Tae•nia
 T. saginata
 T. solium

tae•nia *pl.* tae•niae
 taeniae coli
 t. libera
 t. mesocolica
 t. omentalis
 taeniae pylori
 taeniae of Valsalva

tae•ni•a•sis

tag
 hemorrhoidal t.
 posterior sentinel t.
 rectal t.

Tag•a•met

tail
 t. of pancreas

Tal•ma
 Stokvis-T. syndrome

TAM
 tamoxifen

Tam
 tamoxifen

ta•mox•i•fen

tam•pon•ade
 balloon t.
 esophagogastric t.
 ferromagnetic t.

Tan•ner
 T's operation

tape
 ColoScreen t.
 lap t.
 Montgomery's t's
 Transpore t.
 wet t.

Ta•per•cut nee•dle

tape•worm
 armed t.
 beef t.
 fish t.
 pork t.
 unarmed t.

TATA
 transanal abdominal transanal proctosigmoidectomy
 transanal abdominal transanal proctosigmoidectomy and coloanal anastomosis

tau•rine

tau•ro•cho•lan•er•e•sis

tau•ro•cho•lano•poi•e•sis

tau•ro•cho•late

tau•ro•de•oxy•cho•late

tau•ro•hyo•de•oxy•cho•lic

tau•ro•litho•cho•late

tau•ro•ur•so•de•oxy•cho•late

Tay•lor
Herman-T. gastroscope

Taz•i•cef

Taz•i•dime

T bili
total bilirubin

TDMS
tropical diarrhea-malabsorption syndrome

TE
tracheoesophageal

tear
Mallory-Weiss t.

Teb•a•mide

Techne•Coll

Techne•Scan HIDA

Techne•Scan MAA

Techne•Scan PYP

tech•ne•ti•um
t. Tc 99m albumin aggregated
t. Tc 99m disofenin
t. Tc 99m lidofenin
t. Tc 99m mebrofenin
t. Tc 99m PYP
t. Tc 99m pyrophosphate
t. Tc 99m (pyro- and trimeta-) phosphates
t. Tc 99m sulfur colloid

tech•nique
antecolic t.
anterior t.
antiperistaltic t.
Babcock t.
Balfour t.
Braun and Jaboulay t.
coaxial introducing t.
Colp-Hofmeister t.
combined abdominal transsacral resection t.
continuous pull-out t.

tech•nique *(continued)*
Ferguson t.
guillotine t.
Hofmeister-Finsterer t.
Horsley t.
hot-biopsy forceps t.
"hot squeeze" t.
Jaboulay t.
Judd t.
Latzko t.
lift and cut t.
Menghini t.
Mikulicz t.
Moynihan t.
mucosal relief t.
no-touch t.
no-touch isolation t.
Ogilvie t.
overtube-endoscope t.
paintbrush t.
paracoccygeal t.
Polya t., anterior
Polya t., posterior
Ponsky-Gauderer t.
pull-through t.
Russell t.
Sacks-Vine t.
Schoemaker-Billroth II t.
station pull-through t.
transsphincteric t.
trocar t.
Tru-Cut t.
two-scope t.
Vim-Silverman t.
von Haberer-Finney t.
Wangensteen t.
Zieman t.

TEF
tracheoesophageal fistula

Tef•lon cath•e•ter

Tef•lon ERCP can•nu•la

teg•a•fur

Teg•a•mide

te•la *pl.* te•lae
t. submucosa coli

te•la *(continued)*
t. submucosa esophagi
t. submucosa gastris
t. submucosa intestini tenuis
t. submucosa oesophagi
t. submucosa recti
t. submucosa ventriculi
t. subserosa coli
t. subserosa gastris
t. subserosa hepatis
t. subserosa intestini tenuis
t. subserosa peritonei
t. subserosa ventriculi
t. subserosa vesicae biliaris
t. subserosa vesicae felleae

tel•an•gi•ec•ta•sia
gastric t.
hereditary hemorrhagic t.
nonhereditary hemorrhagic t.

Tele•paque

tele•scope
Wolff t.

Tem•po

te•nas•cin

ten•der•ness
rebound t.

ten•do *pl.* ten•di•nes
t. cricoesophageus

ten•don
cricoesophageal t.

te•nes•mus
rectal t.

te•ni•a•my•ot•o•my

1090 Ga•vage Bag

TEN tube feed•ing for•mu•la

te•ra•to•ma *pl.* te•ra•to•mas, te•ra•to•ma•ta

te•ra•to•ma *(continued)*
sacrococcygeal dermoid t.

Ter•ra•my•cin

Ter•ri•er
Courvoisier-T. syndrome

test
acid-clearing t.
acid reflux t.
acid-stripping t.
aminopyrine breath t.
augmented histamine t.
augmented secretin t.
balloon-retaining t.
basal gastric secretion t.
benzidine t.
Bernstein t.
bilirubin t.
Bozicevich's t.
breath t.
Bromsulphalein t.
Bromsulphalein retention t.
BTP (*N*-benzoyl-L-tyrosyl-f-aminobenzoic acid) t.
Bz-Ty-PABA t.
cholyl ^{14}Cr-glycine t.
ColoCARE fecal occult blood t.
ColoScreen fecal occult blood t.
^{14}Cr-aminopyrine breath t.
^{14}Cr-diazepam breath t.
^{14}Cr-galactose breath t.
^{14}Cr-phenacetin breath t.
double-labeled Schilling t.
Einhorn string t.
esophageal acid infusion t.
esophageal provocation t.
fecal occult blood t.
flocculation t.
Fouchet's t.
fructose tolerance t.
galactose breath t.
galactose elimination t.
gastric function t.
glucose tolerance t.

test *(continued)*
- glutoid t.
- Gluzinski's t.
- glycyltryptophan t.
- Graham's t.
- Gross' t.
- Günzberg's t.
- Hamel's t.
- Hay's t.
- Hemoccult t.
- hemoglobin t.
- hepatic function t.
- Histalog t.
- histamine t.
- Hoesch t.
- Hollander's t.
- Huppert's t.
- Huppert-Cole t.
- hydrogen breath t.
- indocyanine green t.
- insulin hypoglycemia t.
- intraductal secretin t. (IDST)
- Javorski's (Jaworski's) t.
- Kashiwado's t.
- Kelling's t.
- Kinberg's t.
- lactose tolerance t.
- latex fixation t.
- levulose tolerance t.
- lipase t.
- liver function t.
- Lundh t.
- Macdonald's t.
- MacLean t.
- Maly's t.
- maximal stimulation t.
- maximum acid output t.
- methemalbumin t.
- methyl red t.
- Mett's t.
- Mohr's t.
- Moynihan's t.
- Murphy's t.
- Myers and Fine t.
- Mylius' t.
- Nakayama's t.
- Neubauer and Fischer's t.

test *(continued)*
- Neukomm's t.
- nitrogen partition t.
- occult blood t.
- PABA (para-aminobenzoic acid) t.
- palmin t.
- palmitin t.
- pancreatic function t.
- peak acid output t.
- pentane breath t.
- phenoltetrachlorophthalein t.
- pineapple t.
- quantitative fecal fat t.
- Quick's t.
- Rehfuss' t.
- Robinson-Kepler-Power water t.
- rose bengal t.
- rose bengal sodium iodine-131 t.
- Rosenbach-Gmelin t.
- Rosenthal's t.
- Sahli's t.
- Sahli's glutoid t.
- Sahli-Nencki t.
- saline infusion t.
- Salkowski and Schipper's t.
- salol t.
- santonin t.
- Schilling t.
- Schumm's t.
- screening t.
- secretin t.
- Seidlitz powder t.
- serum amylase t.
- serum gastrin t.
- Smith's t.
- Stokvis' t.
- Stoll t.
- Sudan III t.
- sulfobromophthalein t.
- Szabo's t.
- Töpfer's t's
- Torquay's t.
- Tuttle t.

test *(continued)*
- Uffelmann's t.
- urea breath t.
- Voges-Proskauer t.
- von Jaksch's t.
- Wagner's t.
- water-gurgle t.
- Watson-Schwartz t.
- Winckler t.
- Witz's t.
- Woldman's t.
- Wolff-Junghans t.
- D-xylose absorption t.
- D-xylose tolerance t.
- Zappacosta's t.

test•ing
- ambulatory manometric t.
- fecal occult blood t.
- standard acid reflux t. (SART)

test meal
- Boyden t. m.

Tes•u•loid

tet•ra•chlo•ro•eth•ane

tet•ra•cy•cline

Tet•ra•cyn

tet•ra•pep•tide

tet•ra•pren•yl•ac•e•tone

tet•ra•zo•li•um
- nitroblue t.

Tev•dek suture

TF
- tube feeding

TG
- thioguanine
- triglyceride

Tg
- thioguanine

6-Tg
- 6-thioguanine

T-Gen

Thal
- T. esophagogastrostomy

Thay•sen
- Gee-T. disease
- T's disease

Theile
- T's glands

Theis
- T. self-retaining retractor

the•o•ry
- overflow t.

Ther•a•lax

ther•a•py
- ablative laser t.
- bile acid t.
- branched-chain amino acid t.
- diet t.
- drug t.
- endoscopic t.
- endoscopic laser t. (ELT)
- enterostomal t.
- hormone t.
- injection t.
- laser t.
- massage t.
- mechanical t.
- photodynamic t.
- protein-calorie t.
- replacement t.
- scleral t.
- thermal t.
- topical t.
- ultrasonic t.

Ther•evac Plus

Ther•evac-SB

thi•a•mine

thio•gua•nine

thi•ol
- protein t.

Thiry
T.-Vella fistula

Tho•mas
Dixon-T.-Smith colon clamp

Thoms
T.-Allis tissue forceps

Tho•rek
T. dissecting scissors
T. gallbladder aspirator
T.-Mixter gallbladder forceps

Tho•ro•trast

Thow
T. tube

thre•o•nine

throm•bo•sis
hepatic vein t.

throm•bus *pl.* throm•bi
bile t.

thumb•print•ing

ti•azo•fur•in

Ti•car

ti•car•cil•lin
t. and clavulanate

Ti•con

Ti-Cron su•ture

tide
alkaline t.

tie
plain catgut t.
silk t.

Ti•gan

Ti•ja

Ti•ject-20

time
acid clearance t.
bleeding t.

time *(continued)*
chromoscopy t.
dextrinizing t.
gut transit t.

Ti•men•tin

tinc•ture
opium t.

ti•nid•a•zole

tip
contact probe t.
lateral prismatic probe t.
sapphire probe t.
suction t.

tis•sue
esophagophrenic t.
extraperitoneal t.
granulation t.
gut-associated lymphoid t. (GALT)
hemorrhoidal t.
right gutter t.

Ti•trac•id

Ti•tra•lac

Tit•ra•lac Plus

TMCA

TNM
tumor-node-metastasis

to•bra•my•cin

Todd
T's cirrhosis

Toep•fer
T's reagent

tol•bu•ta•mide

Tol•er•ex tube feed•ing for•mu•la

Tom Jones
T.J. closure
T.J. near-and-far suture

to•mog•ra•phy
  computed t.
  quantitative computed t.

tone
  rectal t.
  resting anal t.

tongue

to•nom•e•try

Töp•fer
  T's tests

Top-Fill en•ter•al feed•ing bag

To•rek
  T. operation

tor•mi•na

tor•mi•nal

Tor•quay
  T's test

To•ta•cil•lin

touch
  rectal t.

tox•in
  botulinum A t.
  Clostridium difficile t.
  Shiga t.

TPC
  total proctocolectomy

TPN
  total parenteral nutrition

tract
  alimentary t.
  biliary t.
  digestive t.
  fistulous t.
  gastrointestinal t.
  granulating t.
  intestinal t.
  pancreaticobiliary t.

train•ing
  bowel t.

Tral Film•tabs

trans•am•i•nase

Trans•derm-Scōp

Trans•derm-V

trans•glu•tam•in•ase

trans•il•lu•mi•na•tion

tran•sit
  colonic t.
  gastrointestinal (GI) t.
  intestinal t.

trans•pap•il•lary

trans•plant
  Gallie t.

trans•plan•ta•tion
  hepatocyte t.
  liver t.
  orthotopic liver t.
  small bowel t.

Trans•pore tape

trans•port
  hepatocellular t.
  ion t.
  nutrient t.
  sodium-coupled hepatic t.
  sodium-hexose t.
  vesicular t.

trans•po•si•tion
  gluteus maximus t.

trans•va•te•ri•an

Trask
  T. colostomy dome

Trau•ma•Cal tube feed•ing for•mu•la

Traum-Aid HBC stress for•mu•la

Trav•a•sorb feed•ing tube

Trav•a•sorb he•pat•ic di•et

Trav•a•sorb HN tube feed•ing for•mu•la

Trav•a•sorb MCT tube feed•ing for•mu•la

Trav•a•sorb pro•tein and cal•o•rie sup•ple•ment

Trav•a•sorb re•nal di•et

Trav•a•sorb STD tube feed•ing for•mu•la

Trav•a•sorb tube feed•ing for•mu•la

Travenol en•ter•al feed•ing con•tain•er

treat•ment
  Sippy t.

Treitz
  T's fossa
  T's hernia
  T's ligament
  T's muscle

Tren•del•en•burg
  T. position

Treves
  T's fold

tri•ad
  Charcot's t.
  Dieulafoy's t.
  hepatic t's
  portal t's
  Saint's t.
  t. of Schultz

Tri•ad•a•pin

tri•ad•i•tis
  portal t.

tri•an•gle
  Calot's t.
  cystohepatic t.
  Grynfeltt's t.
  t. of Grynfeltt and Lesgaft
  Lesgaft's t.
  Livingston's t.

tri•an•gle *(continued)*
  mesenteric t.

tri•az•i•nate

Tri•a•zole

Tri•ban

Tri•ben•za•gan

Trich•i•nel•la
  T. spiralis

trich•i•no•sis

tri•chlo•ro•eth•y•lene

tricho•be•zoar

Trich•o•mo•nas
  T. hominis

tricho•phy•to•be•zoar

trich•u•ri•a•sis

Trich•u•ris
  T. trichiura

Tri•con•sil

tri•di•hex•eth•yl

tri•glyc•er•ide
  long-chain t.
  medium-chain t. (MCT)
  short-chain t.

Tri•ka•cide

Tri•lax

Tri•ma•deau
  T's sign

Tri•ma•zide

tri•meth•o•ben•za•mide

tri•meth•o•prim
  sulfamethoxazole and t.

Tri•meth-Sul•fa

tri•me•trex•ate

tri•mip•ra•mine

Tri•mox

Trim•pex

tri•pep•tide

Tri•sul•fam

tro•car
- Allen cecostomy t.
- Beardsley cecostomy t.
- intestinal decompression t.
- Ochsner gallbladder t.

T-rod

Troi•sier
- T's node

Tru-Cut tech•nique

trun•cus *pl.* trun•ci
- t. coeliacus
- trunci intestinales
- t. vagalis anterior
- t. vagalis posterior

trunk
- celiac t.
- intestinal t's
- vagal t.
- vagal t., anterior
- vagal t., posterior

truss

try•pano•ci•dal

try•pano•cide

Try•pan•o•so•ma
- *T. cruzi*

try•pano•so•mal

try•pano•some

try•pano•so•mi•ci•dal

try•pano•so•mi•cide

tryp•sin

tryp•tase

tryp•to•phan

TSC

TTS ("through the scope") di•la•tor

T-tube
- T-t. cholangiogram
- T-t. drainage

tube
- Abbott-Miller t.
- Abbott-Rawson t.
- Adson suction t.
- All-Silicone Side-Eye EFT feeding t.
- Bilboa-Dotter t.
- Cantor t.
- Cattell T-t.
- C-Flex t.
- Chaffin sump t.
- t. clogging
- Coloshield t.
- Corsafe feeding t.
- Davol colon t.
- Davol feeding t.
- Diamond's t.
- digestive t.
- Dobbhoff feeding t.
- double-lumen t.
- Dreiling t.
- Dumon-Gilliard prosthesis pushing t.
- Duo-Tube feeding t.
- Edlich t.
- Endo-Tube feeding t.
- enterostomy t.
- Entriflex feeding t.
- Entri-HN feeding t.
- ENtube feeding t.
- ENtube Plus feeding t.
- ENtube-Pedi feeding t.
- esophageal t.
- Ethox feeding t.
- Ewald t.
- feeding t.
- Flexi-Flow feeding t.
- FlowThruEFT feeding t.
- flushing t.
- Frederick Miller feeding t.
- gastronomy t.
- gastrostomy t.
- Gilman-Abrams gastric t.
- Harris t.

tube *(continued)*
Hemovac t.
intracolonic bypass t.
jejunostomy t.
Johnson intestinal t.
K-t.
Kaslow plastic stomach irrigation t.
Kehr's T-t.
Keofeed II feeding t.
t. kinking
Levin t.
Levin duodenal t.
McLean-Ring feeding t.
Medovations feeding t.
Miller rectal t.
Miller-Abbott t.
Miller-Abbott double-lumen t.
Miller-Abbott intestinal t.
Nachlas gastrointestinal t.
nasoenteric t.
nasogastric t.
nonweighted t.
Ochsner gallbladder t.
Panda feeding t.
Paul-Mixter t.
pediatric feeding t.
pharyngostomy t.
polyurethane t.
polyvinylchloride (PVC) t.
Poole suction t.
pusher t.
Rehfuss' t.
Rehfuss' duodenal t.
Rubin-Quinton small bowel biopsy t.
Ryle's t.
Ryle's duodenal t.
Sengstaken-Blakemore t.
Shiner's t.
Silastic t.
silicone t.
silicone elastomer t.
silicone rubber t.
Silk Bullet feeding t.
Silk Pill feeding t.
Silk Tip feeding t.

tube *(continued)*
stomach t.
suction t.
T-t.
tampon t.
Thow t.
Travasorb feeding t.
triple-lumen t.
Wangensteen t.
Waters t.
weighted t.
Yankauer suction t.

tu•ber *pl.* tu•bers, tu•be•ra
t. omentale hepatis
t. omentale pancreatis
omental t. of liver
omental t. of pancreas
papillary t. of liver

tu•ber•cle
caudal t. of liver
papillary t.

tu•ber•cu•lo•sis

tu•bule
biliferous t.

tu•bu•lo•ves•i•cle

tu•bu•lo•ve•sic•u•lar

tu•bu•lo•vil•lous

tu•bu•lus *pl.* tu•bu•li
t. biliferus

tu•bus *pl.* tu•bi
t. digestorius

Tuck•er
T. dilator

Tuf•fier
T's inferior ligament

Tul•pi•us
valve of T.

tu•meur
t. pileuse

tu•mor
aggressive t.

tu•mor *(continued)*
carcinoid t.
desmoid t.
exophytic t.
fecal t.
gastric t.
glomus t.
Krukenberg's t.
mesenteric desmoid t.
polypoid t.
rectal carcinoid t.
stercoral t.
ulcerated t.
Zollinger-Ellison (ZE) t.

tu•mor•i•gen•e•sis

Tums

tu•nic
fibrous t. of liver

tu•ni•ca *pl.* tu•ni•cae
t. adventitia esophagi
t. adventitia oesophagi
t. fibrosa hepatis
t. mucosa coli
t. mucosa esophagi
t. mucosa gastris
t. mucosa intestini recti
t. mucosa intestini tenuis
t. mucosa oesophagi
t. mucosa recti
t. mucosa ventriculi
t. mucosa vesicae biliaris
t. mucosa vesicae felleae
t. muscularis coli
t. muscularis esophagi
t. muscularis gastris
t. muscularis intestini tenuis
t. muscularis oesophagi
t. muscularis recti
t. muscularis ventriculi
t. muscularis vesicae biliaris
t. muscularis vesicae felleae
t. serosa coli
t. serosa gastris

tu•ni•ca *(continued)*
t. serosa hepatis
t. serosa intestini tenuis
t. serosa peritonei
t. serosa ventriculi
t. serosa vesicae biliaris
t. serosa vesicae felleae

Turck
T's zone

Tur•cot
T. syndrome

tu•ris•ta

Turn•bull
T. blow-hole procedure

Tur•ner
T's sign

Tu•rell
T. angulated specimen forceps
T. proctoscope
T. sigmoidoscope

Tut•tle
T's proctoscope
T. sigmoidoscope
T. test

Ty•cron su•ture

tym•pan•ia

tym•pa•nism

tym•pa•ni•tes

tym•pa•nit•ic

tym•pa•ny

typh•lec•ta•sis

typh•lec•to•my

typh•lo•dic•li•di•tis

typh•lo•pexy

typh•los•to•my

typh•lot•o•my

ty•ro•pa•no•ate so•di•um

ty•ro•sine

ty•ro•sine am•i•no•trans•fer•ase

ty•ro•sin•emia
hereditary t.
persistent t.
transitory t.

U

UBW
usual body weight

UC
ulcerative colitis

UDC
ursodeoxycholate

UDCA
ursodeoxycholic acid

UES
upper esophageal sphincter

UFA
unesterified fatty acids

Uf•fel•mann
U's test

UGI
upper gastrointestinal

UGI se•ries

UGI se•ries with small bow•el fol•low-through

UICC
Union Internationale Contre Cancer

UIQ
upper inner quadrant

ul•cer
anal u.
anastomotic u.
aphthous u.
Barrett's u.
bleeding u.
coalescent u's
u. collar
collar button u.
u. crater
Cruveilhier's u.
Cushing's u.
Cushing-Rokitansky u.

ul•cer *(continued)*
Dieulafoy's u.
duodenal u.
esophageal u.
flask u.
gastric u.
giant peptic u's
girdle u.
jejunal u.
kissing u's
Kocher's dilatation u.
linear u.
marginal u.
u. mound
peptic u.
pyloric channel u.
rectal u.
Rokitansky-Cushing u's
round u.
sea anemone u.
secondary jejunal u.
stercoraceous u.
stercoral u.
stoma u.
stomal u.
stress u.

ul•cer•at•ed

ul•cer•a•tion
acute stress u.
peristomal u.

ul•cus *pl.* ul•ce•ra
u. ventriculi

ULQ
upper left quadrant

ul•tra•so•nog•ra•phy
endoscopic u.
intraluminal u.
intrarectal u.

ul•tra•sound
endoscopic u.
transrectal u.

Ul•tra-Tech•ne•Kow

um•bil•i•co•por•tog•ra•phy

Una•syn

Uni•pen

unit
  Bovie electrosurgical u.
  Cameron electrosurgical u.
  Cameron-Miller electrocoagulation u.
  electrosurgical u.
  endoscopy u.
  Philips RT50 radiotherapy u.
  Valleylab E3B cautery u.
  Valleylab SSE2-K electrosurgery u.

Uni•ted Os•to•my As•so•ci•a•tion (UOA)

Uni•vol

UOA
  United Ostomy Association

UOQ
  upper outer quadrant

UQ
  upper quadrant

Ura•beth

urea

Ure•cho•line

uro•bi•lin

uro•bi•lino•gen
  urine u.

urog•ra•phy
  intravenous u.

uro•ki•nase

Uro•plus

uro•por•phy•rin•o•gen de•car•boxy•lase

URQ
  upper right quadrant

ur•so•de•oxy•cho•late

ur•so•de•oxy•cho•lic acid

ur•so•di•ol

Ush•er
  U.-Bellis hernia repair

U.S. re•trac•tor

UUN
  urine urea nitrogen

V

V
  vomiting

VA
  villous adenoma

vac•cine
  hepatitis B v.

va•got•o•my
  bilateral v.
  highly selective v.
  medical v.
  parietal cell v.
  proximal gastric v.
  selective v.
  supradiaphragmatic v.
  surgical v.
  transthoracic v.
  truncal v.

val•ine

val•le•cu•la *pl.* val•le•cu•lae
  v. ovata

Val•ley•lab E3B cau•tery unit

val•pro•ic ac•id

Val•sal•va
  taeniae of V.

val•va *pl.* val•vae
  v. ilealis
  v. ileocaecalis

valve
  anal v's
  Ball's v's
  ball v.
  Bauhin's v.
  fallopian v.
  Gerlach's v.
  Heister's v.
  Houston's v's
  ileocecal v.
  ileocolic v.
  Kerckring's v's

valve *(continued)*
  Kohlrausch's v's
  v. of Macalister
  Morgagni's v's
  nipple v.
  O'Beirne's v.
  pyloric v.
  semilunar v's of colon
  semilunar v's of Morgagni
  sigmoid v's of colon
  spiral v. of cystic duct
  spiral v. of Heister
  v. of Tulpius
  v. of Varolius
  v. of vermiform appendix

val•vu•la *pl.* val•vu•lae
  valvulae anales
  valvulae conniventes
  v. ileocolica
  v. processus vermiformis
  v. pylori
  v. spiralis [Heisteri]

Van•co•cin

Van•co•led

van•co•my•cin

Van•cor

van Cre•veld
  Ellis-van C. syndrome

van den Bergh
  van den B's disease

Var•co
  Dennis and V. operation
  V. gallbladder forceps

var•i•ce•al

var•i•ces

var•ix *pl.* var•i•ces
  downhill varices
  esophageal v.
  gastric v.

var•ix *(continued)*
  mesenteric v.

Va•ro•li•us
  valve of V.

vas *pl.* va•sa
  vasa aberrantis hepatis

Va•se•line gauze pack

Va•se•line gauze plug

Va•se•line gauze strip

vaso•pres•sin

Va•ter
  ampulla of V.
  papilla of V.

va•ter•i•an seg•ment

VBL
  vinblastine

Vbl
  vinblastine

VCR
  vincristine

Vcr
  vincristine

vec•tog•ra•phy
  anal pressure v.

veil
  Jackson's v.

vein
  Burow's v.
  central v's of liver
  colic v., left
  colic v., middle
  colic v., right
  cystic v.
  epigastric v., inferior
  epigastric v., superficial
  epigastric v's, superior
  epiploic v., left
  epiploic v., right
  esophageal v's
  gastric v., left

vein *(continued)*
  gastric v., right
  gastric v's, short
  gastroepiploic v., left
  gastroepiploic v., right
  gastro-omental v., left
  gastro-omental v., right
  hemiazygos v.
  hepatic v's
  hepatic v's, left
  hepatic v's, middle
  hepatic v's, right
  ileocolic v.
  jejunal v's
  Krukenberg's v's
  mesenteric v.
  mesenteric v., inferior
  mesenteric v., superior
  pancreatic v's
  pancreaticoduodenal v's
  paraumbilical v's
  portal v.
  prepyloric v.
  rectal v's, inferior
  rectal v's, middle
  rectal v., superior
  Retzius's v's
  sigmoid v's
  splenic v.
  subcostal v.
  submucosal v.

Vel•ban

Vel•la
  V. fistula

Vel•peau
  V's hernia

ve•na *pl.* ve•nae
  v. cava inferior
  venae centrales hepatis
  v. colica dextra
  v. colica intermedia
  v. colica media
  v. colica sinistra
  v. cystica
  v. epigastrica inferior
  v. epigastrica superficialis

ve•na *(continued)*
- venae epigastricae superiores
- v. epiploica dextra
- v. epiploica sinistra
- venae gastricae breves
- v. gastrica dextra
- v. gastrica sinistra
- v. gastroepiploica dextra
- v. gastroepiploica sinistra
- v. gastro-omentalis dextra
- v. gastro-omentalis sinistra
- venae hepaticae
- venae hepaticae dextrae
- venae hepaticae intermediae
- venae hepaticae mediae
- venae hepaticae sinistrae
- v. ileocolica
- inferior v. cava
- venae jejunales
- v. mesenterica inferior
- v. mesenterica superior
- venae oesophageales
- venae pancreaticae
- venae pancreaticoduodenales
- venae paraumbilicales
- v. portae hepatis
- v. portalis hepatis
- v. prepylorica
- venae rectales inferiores
- venae rectales mediae
- v. rectalis superior
- venae sigmoideae
- v. splenica
- v. subcostalis
- superior v. cava

ve•nog•ra•phy
- hepatic v.
- portal v.

ven•tric•u•li

ven•tric•u•lus *pl.* ven•tric•u•li

ven•trop•to•sia

ven•trop•to•sis

ven•ule
- submucosal v.

ver•ap•a•mil

verge
- anal v.

ver•mic•u•la•tion

ver•mix

Ver•ner
- V.-Morrison syndrome

Ver•non
- V.-David proctoscope
- V.-David rectal speculum
- V.-David sigmoidoscope

Ver•res
- V. needle

ver•ru•ca *pl.* ver•ru•cae
- anal v.

Ver•sa•bran

ve•si•ca *pl.* ve•si•cae
- v. biliaris
- v. fellea

ves•i•cle
- biliary v.
- brush border membrane v.
- liposomal v.

ve•sic•u•la *pl.* ve•sic•u•lae
- v. bilis
- v. fellea

ves•sel
- bile v.
- hemorrhoidal v's
- hypogastric v.
- left colic v.
- nonbleeding visible v.
- omphalomesenteric v.

ves•ti•bule
- v. of omental bursa

ves•tib•u•lum *pl.* ves•tib•u•la
- v. bursae omentalis

V-Gan

VH
viral hepatitis

VHDL
very-high-density lipoprotein

Vi•bra•my•cin

Vib•rio
V. alginolyticus
V. cholerae
V. cholerae biotype *albensis*
V. cholerae biotype *cholerae*
V. cholerae biotype *eltor*
V. cholerae biotype *proteus*
V. eltor
V. fluvialis
V. furnissii
V. hollisae
V. metschnikovii
V. parahaemolyticus
V. vulnificus

vib•rio *pl.* vib•rios or vib•ri•o•nes
Celebes v.
cholera v.
El Tor v.
v. group EF-6
v. group F
NAG v's
nonagglutinating v's
noncholera v's
paracholera v's

vib•rio•ci•dal

Vi•cryl su•ture

Vi•deo•En•do•scope sys•tem

vi•deo•en•dos•co•py

vil•lous

vil•lus *pl.* vil•li
intestinal villi
villi intestinales

vil•lus *(continued)*
villi of small intestine

Vim
V.-Silverman needle
V.-Silverman technique

vi•men•tin

vin•blas•tine

Vin•ca•sar

Vin•crex

vin•cris•tine

vin•de•sine

Vine
Sacks-V. technique

Vin•son
Plummer-V. syndrome

vi•nyl
v. chloride

Vi•o•kase pancreatic enzymes

VIP
vasoactive intestinal polypeptide

Vir•chow
V's node

vi•rus
hepatitis v.
hepatitis A v. (HAV)
hepatitis B v. (HBV)
hepatitis C v. (HCV)
hepatitis delta v.
human immunodeficiency v. (HIV)
Norwalk v.

vis•ce•ra
abdominal v.

Vis•cer•ol

vis•cero•tome

vis•cer•ot•o•my

vis•cos•i•ty
bile v.

Vis•ta•ject

Vis•ta•ril

Vis•ta•zine

Vi•tal tube feed•ing for•mu•la

vi•ta•min
v. A
v. B_1
v. B_2
v. B_6
v. B_{12}
v. C
v. D
v. E
fat-soluble v's
v. K
water-soluble v's

Vi•ta•need tube feed•ing for•mu•la

Vi•vo•nex Acu•trol En•ter•al Feed•ing Sys•tem

Vi•vo•nex pro•tein and cal•o•rie sup•ple•ment

Vi•vo•nex TEN stress for•mu•la

V-Lax

VLDL
very-low-density lipoprotein

β-VLDL
β-very-low-density lipoprotein

Voges
V.-Proskauer test

Volk•mann
V. rake retractor
V. retractor

vol•ume
gastric v.
stool v.

vol•vu•late

vol•vu•lus
cecal v.
colonic v.
gastric v.
v. neonatorum
sigmoid v.
transverse colon v.

vom•it
bilious v.
black v.
coffee-ground v.

vom•it•ing
cyclic v.
dry v.
fecal v.
hysterical v.
periodic v.
projectile v.
recurrent v.
stercoraceous v.

vom•it•u•ri•tion

vom•i•tus
v. cruentus
v. matutinus

von Gier•ke
von G's disease

von Ha•ber•er
von H.-Finney technique

von Jaksch
von J's test

von Kupf•fer
von K's cells

von Mer•ing
von M. reflex

von Mey•er•berg
von M. complexes

von Petz
  von P. clamp
  von P. sewing machine
  von P. stomach clamp
  von P. suture clip
  von P. suturing apparatus

Von•trol

VP-16
  etoposide

Vp-16
  etoposide

V sign of Na•cle•rio

VTR-300 en•ter•al feed•ing pump

V-Y ano•plas•ty

W

wa•fer
Stomahesive w.

Wag•ner
W's test

Wal•dey•er
W's fascia
W's fossa

Wales
W. rectal bougie

Walk•er
Osler-W.-Rendu syndrome
W. gallbladder retractor

wall
belly w.

Wan•gen•steen
W. anastomosis clamp
W's apparatus
W. drainage
W. suction
W. suction apparatus
W. technique
W. tube

WAR
whole abdominal radiotherapy

War•ren
W. shunt

War•then
W. spur crusher

War•thin
W.-Starry stain

wash•out
high colonic w.
rectal w.

Was•ko
W. common duct probe

wa•ter brash

wa•ter jet

Wa•ters
W. tube

Wat•son
W.-Schwartz test

Watts
W. locking clamp

Waugh
W. and Clagett operation

wave
cat w's

wave•guide
flexible quartz w.

WDHA
watery diarrhea with hypokalemic alkalosis

WDHH
watery diarrhea, hypokalemia, and hypovolemia

web
esophageal w.
intestinal w.

weight
actual w. (AW)
actual body w. (ABW)
ideal body w. (IBW)
usual body w.

Wein•berg
W. retractor

Weir
Fowler-W. incision

Weiss
Mallory-W. laceration
Mallory-W. syndrome
Mallory-W. tear

Weit•lan•er
W. retractor

Welch Al•lyn fi•ber•op•tic proc•to•scope

Welch Al•lyn 80055 fi•ber•op•tic sig•moido•scope

Welch Al•lyn proc•to•scope

Welch Al•lyn rec•tal hook

Welch Al•lyn rec•tal set

Welch Al•lyn sig•moido•scope

Welch Al•lyn vi•deo co•lono•scope

Welch Al•lyn vi•deo en•do•scope

Well•co•vo•rin

Well•fe•ron

Wells
W. procedure
W. thumb tissue forceps

Wert•heim
W. pedicle clamp

Whip•ple
W's disease
W's operation

whip•worm

White
Winsbury-W. deep retractor

White•head
modified W. hemorrhoidectomy
W's operation

Whit•more
W. bag

Wil•lau•er
W. thoracic scissors

Wil•li
Prader-W. syndrome

Wil•liams
W. intestinal forceps
W. overtube sleeve
W. tissue forceps

Wil•lis
antrum of W.
W's pancreas
W. pouch

Wil•son
W. torque guide

Wil•son-Cook en•do•pros•the•sis

Wil•son-Cook litho•trip•tor

Winck•ler
W. test

Win•Gel

Wins•bury
W.-White deep retractor

Wins•low
foramen of W.
hiatus of W.
W's pancreas

Win•tro•cin

wire
cautery w.
stainless steel w.

Wir•sung
canal of W.
duct of W.

Witz
W's test

Wit•zel
W. closure
W. gastrostomy
W's operation

Wold•man
W's test

Wolf
W.-Schindler gastroscope

Wolff
W.-Junghans test

Wolff tele•scope

Wölf•ler
W's operation

Wolf•son
DeMartel-W. anastomosis clamp
DeMartel-W. clamp
DeMartel-W. clamp holder
DeMartel-W. closing forceps
Percy-W. retractor
W. gallbladder retractor

Wol•man
W's disease

Wood
Crile-W. needle holder

Wood•ward
W. esophagogastrostomy

Wor•rall
W. deep retractor

wrap•ping
fundic w.

Wut•zer
W. hernia

Wya•my•cin-E

Wya•my•cin-S

Wy•mox

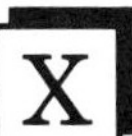

xan•thine de•hy•dro•gen•ase

xan•thine ox•i•dase

xan•tho•ma
  gastric x.

X-Prep Li•quid

xy•lose

Y

Yan•kau•er
Y. suction tube

Yeo•mans
Y. proctoscope
Y. rectal biopsy forceps
Y. sigmoidoscope

Yer•sin•ia
Y. enterocolitica
Y. frederiksenii

Yer•sin•ia (continued)
Y. intermedia
Y. kristensenii
Y. pseudotuberculosis

Y glass rod

Yo•shi-864

Young
Y. tongue forceps

Z

Z line

Zach•a•ry Cope
Z.C.-DeMartel colon clamp

zac•o•pride

Zahn
anomaly of Z.

Zan•ca
Z's syndrome

Zan•tac

Zap•pa•cos•ta
Z's test

Ze•fa•zone

Zeis•sel
Z's layer

Zell•weg•er
Z. syndrome

Zen•ker
Z's pouch

zi•do•vu•dine

Zie•man
Z. technique

zinc
hair z.
nail z.
plasma z.
z. sulfate

zin•o•stat•in

Zix•or•yn

Zol•lin•ger
Z.-Ellison syndrome
Z.-Ellison tumor

zo•na *pl.* zo•nae
z. hemorrhoidalis
z. transformans

zone
hemorrhoidal z.
transformation z.
Turck's z.

zuck•er•guss•darm

zuck•er•guss•le•ber

Zy•mase

Zy•men•ol